Dear Dr. Schwarzbein: Thank you, thank you, thank you. I am fifty-nine years old and have been more or less concerned about good health from the age of twenty-four, following the birth of my second child. Over the years I've done various activities to keep fit—aerobics, walking, swimming, and yoga. And over the years, I continued to gain weight. Six months ago I was going to the gym six days a week and still weighed 150 pounds on a 5'3" frame.

I was very discouraged. Then, someone told me about your book. . . . It has been unbelievable. It's been six months now, and I have lost fifteen pounds, 2½ inches off my waist and the same off my hips. I've gone down two dress sizes. You were so right when you said to throw away the scales. The number doesn't matter; it's what is happening at the metabolic level that counts.

—**Jude,** New Brunswick, Canada

My husband bought *The Schwarzbein Principle* to read for weight loss purposes. Being a registered nurse I scoffed at it. My training is in direct opposition to the idea that one should eat more fat and protein! But after reading Dr. Schwarzbein's introduction to the book, I realized it made sense, so I decided to follow the eating principles for a two-month trial. After just two weeks of eating according to the Principle I was amazed at the physical changes that occurred, which I hadn't known were wrong in the first place! I quit having frequent headaches and feeling shaky before lunch, and I slept much more deeply, almost like the sleep I enjoyed as a child. I am convinced!

—**Carol Feenstra,** Mason, OH

The Schwarzbein Principle has helped me immensely. In the weeks after I began following the book's directives I began to immediately feel better and look better. I dropped two belt sizes and began wearing pants that I had not worn in almost seven years. I have also kept the weight off and no longer crave carbohydrates like I once did. I have also given up caffeine and only occasionally do I sip a glass of wine. Irritable Bowel Syndrome no longer plagues me. I don't know how I put up with that problem for so long! I'm so glad to have found the answer!

—**Paul C.,** Milford, NH

I feel a thousand times better since starting the Schwarzbein Principle—it's great!

—**Leslie Hilton,** Denver, CO

theschwarzbeinprinciple
THE PROGRAM

losing weight the healthy way
an easy, 5-step, no-nonsense approach

Diana Schwarzbein, M.D.

Health Communications, Inc.
Deerfield Beach, Florida

www.bcibooks.com

The Schwarzbein Principle is not intended as a substitute for the advice and/or medical care of the reader's physician, nor is it meant to discourage or dissuade the reader from the advice of his or her physician. The reader should regularly consult with a physician in matters relating to his or her health, and especially with regard to symptoms that may require diagnosis. Any eating or lifestyle regimen should be undertaken under the direct supervision of the reader's physician. Moreover, anyone with chronic or serious ailments should undertake any eating and lifestyle program, and/or changes to his or her personal eating and lifestyle regimen, under the direct supervision of his or her physician. If the reader has any questions concerning the information presented in this book, or its application to his or her particular medical profile, or if the reader has unusual medical or nutritional needs or constraints that may conflict with the advice in this book, he or she should consult his or her physician. If the reader is pregnant or nursing she should consult her physician before embarking on the nutrition and lifestyle program outlined in this book. The reader should not stop prescription medications without the advice and guidance of his or her personal physician.

Library of Congress Cataloging-in-Publication Data

Schwarzbein, Diana, 1960-
    The Schwarzbein principle : the program : losing weight the healthy way : an easy, 5-step, no-nonsense approach / Diana Schwarzbein.
        p. cm.
    ISBN 0-7573-0227-0
    1. Weight loss. 2. Health. 3. Nutrition. I. Title.

RM222.2.S359 2004
613.2'5—dc22

                                                                        2004054274

©2004 Diana Schwarzbein
ISBN 0-7573-0227-0

Publisher: Health Communications, Inc.
          3201 S.W. 15th Street
          Deerfield Beach, FL 33442-8190

Cover design by Larissa Hise Henoch
Inside book design by Lawna Oldfield Patterson
Inside book formatting by Dawn Von Strolley Grove

To Larry,
you are my gravity

Contents

PART III: THE SCHWARZBEIN PLANS

Author's Note

Welcome to *The Schwarzbein Principle: The Program*. In this book, as well as my others, you will learn how your body functions and what you can do to live a long and healthy life. All three books have something to offer you.

I wrote my first book, *The Schwarzbein Principle*, with the goal of getting people to start eating healthy fats again and lower their overall consumption of carbohydrates. This book also helps people conquer their fear of fats.

My second book, *The Schwarzbein Principle II: The Transition*, was written to give you a deeper understanding of the importance of carbohydrates and what you will go through as your metabolism heals. This is where you will find the in-depth scientific explanations behind my program. It is the book to have if you want to know how it all works.

As more people turned to me to help them heal from years of dieting and overexercising, I had to come up with innovative new ways to teach both the public and professionals about my program. The result is this book. *The Schwarzbein Principle: The Program* is the most straightforward approach to following my five-step program as I intend it to be followed. It includes the latest healing and maintenance plans and the most updated information I have to offer. Whether you are already familiar with my program or not, this is the book to have and to follow!

The knowledge in this book is complete and can be applied by anyone. However, if you still want to learn more, I recommend that you read *The Schwarzbein Principle II: The Transition,* and that you visit my Web site at *www.schwarzbeinprinciple.com.*

I look forward to you joining me and thousands of others in the pursuit of optimal health.

Diana Schwarzbein, M.D.

Acknowledgments

The idea for this book is solely the responsibility of Peter Vegso—Peter, be careful what you wish for.

It would never have been started without the enormous help of my sister, Alexis Sersland, and would never have been finished without the immensely talented efforts of Bret Witter, editor extraordinaire, and the staff at HCI, Inc.

More heartfelt thanks go to:

My parents, Martha and Edison Schwarzbein, who are my biggest critics as well as biggest fans. Thanks for the great editing tips. As usual I couldn't have done it without your support. I love you both!

JJ Virgin for her help with the exercise portion of the book and the lifestyle eating tips. You are amazing and I wish you lived closer so that we could accomplish more things together.

Betsy Stanshine for her enormous help with the dietary sections and meal plans. Thanks for the great job.

Mindy Rosenblatt and Evelyn Jacob—two peas in a pod. You were always there when I needed your advice and help. You two are amazing!

Kim Weiss for letting me always call on you whenever I needed help with anything and everything. I want you to know how much you are appreciated.

Eric McFarland for the feedback and all your constructive criticism—it is always welcome and keeps me on my toes! You are the best and I love you dearly, but you will always be shorter.

Sheila Fowler, who likes to see her name in print—thanks for always listening and being such a great long time friend. I love you and wish you were closer.

Mike Bruce and Cathy Ann Simon for their dental expertise.

Rae Lynn Riedel and Randy Bimestefer, it has been great to know you as friends and colleagues. I have enjoyed working with you both. Thanks for all the help.

And the staff of The Schwarzbein Institute, past and present, for putting up with me when I am writing and for all their support:

Chin
Doris Vargas
Jonathan Cooper
Natalie Sanchez
Jay Rohrs
Carol Wilson
Deralee Scanlon
Jane Westerman
Olga Barraza

A special thank you to Suzanne Somers for helping to spread my work. You are a multitalented woman and I feel lucky to have such a great friend and ally as you. And though we don't always agree on the details, we definitely agree on the bigger stuff. Together we are making a difference.

Lastly, I want to personally thank my husband, Larry Mousouris, who is the best thing that ever happened to me as well as the reason that I am able to do as much as I do. You are my rock.

Introduction

To The Schwarzbein Principle Program

A re you looking for a health program that does not require that you starve yourself or exercise all day long to get results? Are you so confused by all the diets out there that you don't know what to believe anymore? Are you at the point in your life that you understand that anything worthwhile takes time and patience to accomplish? Did my first two books leave you wanting a daily, step-by-step planner? If you answered yes to any of these questions, you have picked up the right book.

Welcome to the Schwarzbein Principle, a program designed to help you achieve long-lasting, healthy results. This five-step program prevents damage to your metabolism or helps to heal damage that has already occurred. I promise that if you adopt the SPP as a way of life, you will be healthier, happier and able to achieve your ideal body composition (a balanced amount of lean body tissue and a normal amount of protective fat). Furthermore, once you have healed your metabolism, you will never have to do it again.

Interested? Read on.

Two of the most important principles of my program are that *you need to eat well to build well* and *you need to be healthy to lose weight, not lose weight to be healthy.* If you undereat, eat incorrectly or

overexercise, you will never be healthy because you will be using up your body chemicals faster than you can rebuild them. Whenever you use more than you rebuild, you are aging faster than normal. To slow down the aging process and keep yourself healthier, you will be required to eat more often and exercise less often but more efficiently. By doing so, you enable your body to rebuild and repair itself, which means that you have a healthy metabolism that is primed to help you burn off fat weight without breaking down lean body tissue (muscle and bones).

Sounds too good to be true, right? Well, I want you to know there is plenty of science to back this up.

Damaging Your Metabolism

How does one damage their metabolism? Unfortunately, by following programs that incorporate undereating, eliminating food groups, overexercising, low-fat or low-carbohydrate meal plans, and/or fasting (to name a few bad habits) in order to be "thin" and "healthy." These habits cause changes to your physiology that signal your body to break down. The normal process of aging is due to your body losing its ability to rebuild as well as when you were younger; therefore, any habit that causes you to break down more quickly accelerates aging.

This is how, after years of hard work and deprivation trying to do the "right thing," people become out of shape and sicker than they have ever been. They usually get very frustrated and worn out, too. And worse for some, their fat depositions that used to be evenly distributed all over their body return and localize around their midsection or belly area. They end up with a metabolism so damaged that it no longer responds to undereating and/or overexercising and a body that is aging at a faster rate than it's supposed to. Has this already happened to you? If so, do not despair. As distressing as all this may

be, it is never too late to recognize your past mistakes and make the necessary changes to your nutrition and lifestyle habits to improve your health today.

For those of you who are in the early process of damaging your metabolism it will be harder to understand what I am writing, but think about the following: You cannot feel that you are causing damage while it is happening, only after it has occurred. You become damaged by using up and breaking down your body chemicals and cells. When you are using yourself up, you release energy and other "feel good" chemicals; therefore, the process of breaking down makes you feel more alive. Since it initially feels good doing something that is harmful, you will never think about needing to change your habits. Although you are doing the wrong things, you will still feel as if you are healthy.

For example, you can be following the latest popular craze of not eating enough carbohydrates and you can experience "benefits" such as weight loss, more energy, better mood and lower cholesterol levels. Why is this so terrible? Because it is a short-term fix that will cause damage to your metabolism. By not eating enough carbohydrates, you signal your body to use rather than rebuild. Think of it as your body eating itself up. If you did this on a consistent basis, you would age faster and die younger. Trust me on the physiology.

SPP Is a Health Program

If what I am writing is true, why isn't my program as popular as the Atkins diet? Because I will not, and do not, promote the SPP as a simple weight-loss program. It is a health program. It is hard to compete with all the popular diets promising quick weight loss and everlasting health when my program is offering you everlasting health first and fat weight loss second—*and sometimes a distant second.*

Furthermore, for some of you who have already damaged your

metabolism, healing can involve weight gain. And just like breaking down feels good, healing sometimes feels bad. Try selling that on national TV—a program that could *initially* cause weight gain and *often* makes you feel poorly during the process of healing. Now you can see why my program does not have such widespread appeal. Or why some think my program is crazy. But think about it objectively. My program involves eating balanced meals, managing stress, sleeping through the night, tapering off of toxic chemicals, getting the right amount and kind of exercise, and balancing your body's natural hormones. Which part of this sounds crazy to you?

My program does not tell you what you want to hear. It does not promise falsely that those of you who have damaged your metabolism will feel better instantly or lose fat weight instantaneously. I will not lie to you. And besides, you already know there are no easy answers. If there were a magic pill, you would be taking it already, and I would be prescribing it for you. And if all those years of dieting and over-exercising worked, you wouldn't have picked up this book. You and I both know that it takes time to heal. The good news is that you can still heal by stopping the bad habits that caused you to damage your body in the first place. My program teaches you how.

SPP Is a Process

My program is a process. That is why the five steps have to be followed in a specific order. If you attempt to improve all your habits at the same time, you will rebuild too quickly. You will not be able to handle the symptoms as your body withdraws from its addiction to the breaking down process, and you will always fail this program. It is also why there is a self-medicating phase within the healing phase of the transition. Self-medicating is the process of continuing a bad habit while you improve other habits, thus allowing yourself to feel better as your body begins to repair itself. Self-medicating helps by slowing the

overall rebuilding process because it allows you to continue to break down and use your chemicals to feel better. For some of you who have damaged your metabolism quite severely, self-medicating will be the one thing that will make it possible for you to continue eating well.

What my program ultimately promises is that when you have healed your metabolism, you will be free of destructive habits, feel better than you have in years and have the chance to burn off your excess fat weight.

Informed Choices

You have been lied to. Many of you are trusting that you are getting the correct information to make an intelligent decision on your health choices. But you are not. When you have knowledge that flies in the face of conventional wisdom, as I do, you feel obligated to share it. Once it is out there for you to read and evaluate, my job is finished. If you choose to follow a program *knowing* that you are harming yourself, that is up to you. I believe in the freedom of *informed* choice.

But why does history keep repeating itself? Why have we seen the pendulum swing from a low carbohydrate, high protein/fat diet plan to a high carbohydrate, low protein/fat diet plan and once again back to a low carbohydrate, high protein/fat diet plan? We have already tried all these ways of eating, and if they had worked why would we have changed? The truth is that they don't work. People have become ill and fat from both these ways of eating. Why won't people adopt a more balanced way of eating as promoted in the SPP? The answer is the lure of fast initial results. Later, when the program stops working, most individuals turn the blame back onto themselves. *I could have followed the program better,* they think. Or, *It must have been the few times I cheated that made the whole program not work for me.* This is human nature, and I have heard these same rationalizations from many of my patients when I asked them why they kept up this way of

popular eating when it obviously did not work.

It is time for a paradigm shift, away from thinking that being thin or losing weight will make you healthy to understanding that being healthy will help you stay thin or lose your fat weight. My program is here to help you change your way of thinking.

Helping Thousands to Heal

Why should you believe me? After all, you have probably heard about the other programs by other M.D.s, Ph.D.s and dietitians. What makes my program right? Who am I, and what do I know that they don't know?

My quest for the truth regarding health started after I became seriously ill at age seventeen from years of poor eating habits. Because I was not being helped by conventional wisdom, I started my own research into nutrition and health. Suffice it to say that I had to heal myself from my past habits, and I only succeeded after I got rid of the false notions that it didn't matter what I ate as long as I was thin. Once I was able to overcome this incorrect way of thinking, I was able to obtain optimum health and my ideal body composition.

But the story only begins there. I became so interested in health and nutrition that I decided to go to medical school and become a doctor. After four years of medical school, I spent five more years in post-graduate training and became an endocrinologist. Endocrinology is a specialty of internal medicine that deals with the hormone systems of the body. I learned that hormones control what the body does and that hormones are affected by daily nutrition and lifestyle habits. Once I understood this, everything else fell into place.

I started seeing patients and heard countless stories of poor lifestyle habits, such as skipping meals, eliminating food groups, not getting enough sleep and overexercising. With my background in endocrinology, I was able to understand that all of these poor nutrition and

lifestyle habits would cause hormonal imbalances that lead to chronic illness and/or weight issues. I created my five-step program and began clinical research with patients who had Type II diabetes.

I learned a lot of lessons. The most important one is that it takes a long time to damage your metabolism; therefore, you cannot expect that it will heal overnight. I also learned that no one can be healed with habits that are designed to obtain immediate results in how they feel, or by quick changes in their weight, blood pressure or blood sugar and cholesterol levels. I also found out something about myself. I didn't want to be the type of doctor who treated symptoms with drugs. I wanted to be the physician who taught people how the body works so they could be in control of their own health by choosing to make the necessary changes to their daily nutrition and lifestyle habits.

I admit that I made some mistakes along the way because I initially looked for quick-fix lifestyle changes. But it did not take a long time before I figured out, by seeing what happened to my patients, that quick fixes aren't sustainable.

From the extensive knowledge I gained with my patients with Type II diabetes, it was an easy progression to treating patients with adrenal gland burnout. To this day, I continue to work with patients who have damaged their metabolism with the same poor nutrition and lifestyle habits that you probably have right now, and I have yet to meet any-one who has chronically dieted or overexercised and remained healthy. I don't believe it is possible. In the last 14 years, I have helped thousands of patients turn their health around and experience better health than ever before.

If You Still Don't Believe Me, Just Ask Around

If you still are not convinced, I advise you to speak to sick or over-weight family members and friends. Ask them about their past

nutrition and lifestyle habits. I promise that, just as I have, you will hear stories of chronic dieting or overexercising. You will hear many tales of how people tried to follow calorie-in and calorie-out programs but were unable to keep up with these programs and ended up "falling off" their diets and gaining all the weight back, plus more. Or worse, how while on these programs and following them exactly, they did not get any results. How it used to "work" when they would diet and exercise more, but now they feel hopeless because no matter what they do nothing works!

You will hear women say, "When I look at my pictures from junior high or high school, I wonder why I thought I was so fat. I would give anything to look like that now! Why did I ever start dieting? It was the worst thing I have done to myself."

Or you will hear about those who ended up with depression, asthma, PMS, infertility, or bone loss because they bought into the low-fat movement or followed a vegetarian diet (done incorrectly), all believing this was good for their health.

What I guarantee you won't hear from them are stories of eating balanced meals, managing stress well, sleeping through the night, and avoiding toxic chemicals such as alcohol, diet sodas and sugary foods. Nor will you hear about moderate exercise programs and hormone replacement therapy (HRT). You won't hear these stories because people following a healthy lifestyle designed to balance all the hormones of the body are healthy.

You Can Make a Difference

If you are someone who has damaged your metabolism through poor nutrition and lifestyle habits, please join me. You know you are not overweight or ill because you are genetically inferior or have no will power. You should not be ashamed of how this has happened to you. You need to be part of a grass roots movement that empowers all

of us to stop following popular diets and start learning about balance in our lives. There are millions of you out there who know this and yet your voices are not being heard. Join me now in dispelling this counterproductive myth that *you need to be thin to be healthy.* Many lives are being adversely affected.

I invite you now to become part of the Schwarzbein Principle Program and incorporate the five steps you will be learning about in this book into your life. I know that I can help change your life and health, but you are the one who will be doing all the work by making the necessary changes in your daily habits. I look forward to working with you toward a common goal of health, well-being and ideal body composition.

It is time to get started!

Diana Lynn Schwarzbein, M.D.
www.schwarzbeinprinciple.com

PART I

The Schwarzbein Principle

One

The Schwarzbein Principle

Y ou need to be healthy to lose weight, not lose weight to be healthy. That is the core tenet of my unique weight-loss approach. To explain how important this concept is to your life, I will be brutally honest: If you are following one of the popular diets, whether it is low-carb, low-fat or limited calories, it is killing you. Diets that are designed to get you to lose weight first break down every component of your body. This causes destruction of your metabolic system, and ages everything from your brain cells to your organs to the skin on your face.

If you are overdoing cardiovascular exercise *along with your destructive diet*—such as running, aerobics, kickboxing or spinning—you're killing yourself even faster.

Popular diets and high-impact exercise programs emphasize ways to use up more energy and chemicals than you rebuild. This will cause you to lose weight for a short period of time, but most of the weight loss is due to breaking down cell structures, organ tissue, and muscle and bone tissue, along with fat loss. In essence, you are overstressing and starving your body, forcing it to consume itself to keep you functioning.

Although you initially lose weight on the scale, you will soon find

yourself at a plateau where your body is no longer able to respond to the abuse. It is at this point that your weight will not budge, even if you starve yourself more or exercise harder! Worse yet, by continuing to abuse yourself in the long-term, your body will hit the wall, resulting in accelerated aging, degenerative diseases and more severe symptoms than you had before. This is why so many popular diets end with the *unsuspecting victims*—for lack of a better term—being heavier and less healthy than they were when they started.

There is a solution to this problem. You can lose weight and still have a long, healthy and disease-free life. The key is to embrace the concept that health is more important than weight and to understand that once *you are* healthy, *you can and will* lose weight. Even better, once you are healthy you'll keep that weight off for the rest of your life.

My approach to health is based on metabolic regeneration, the ability to rebuild and repair. Under the right set of conditions, you possess the ability to repair and heal yourself, whether that healing involves weight issues, chemical imbalances, or degenerative diseases of aging in your body. But if you are *not* regenerating, you will *not* have the chemicals that you need to achieve your daily activities or stay healthy. The key to health therefore is to build up your body, not to tear it down.

This is why my health program is different from all the other lifestyle programs being promoted these days. My wellness program focuses on curing all the degenerative diseases of aging, *not just* obesity. This idea is summarized in The Schwarzbein Principle.

The Schwarzbein Principle:
Degenerative diseases of aging are not genetic but acquired. Because the systems of the human body are interconnected, and because one imbalance creates another imbalance, poor eating and lifestyle habits, not genetics, are the major cause of degenerative disease.

The Schwarzbein Principle means that you have more control over your own health and aging than you were led to believe. It is meant to empower you with the knowledge necessary to make the changes to your daily habits that will help determine your own destiny. It does this by reinforcing the concept that your body is connected by chemical reactions and by explaining that what you do on a day-to-day basis will influence how long and how well you live your life.

The Preventable Degenerative Diseases of Aging

Abnormal cholesterol levels

Cancer

Dementia

Depression

Early menopause

Heart disease

High blood pressure

Obesity

Osteoarthritis

Osteoporosis

Stroke

Type II diabetes

The Schwarzbein Principle Program

The Schwarzbein Principle Program works by preventing further damage to your metabolism and helping to heal damage that has already occurred. Years of bad habits—like overexercising and eating the wrong way—can lead to excess weight, illness, disease or simple lack of energy. The good news is that if you take action and change your daily habits, you will be able to reverse or prevent further damage to your body and slow the aging process.

The Schwarzbein Principle Program is a way of life, not a short-term plan, and if followed properly it *will* lead to better health, more vitality and your ideal body composition. Here are the five steps of my program, which we'll talk more about in later chapters:

- **Healthy Nutrition.** There is no calorie counting or meal skipping on the Schwarzbein Principle Program. I encourage you to eat as much as you need up to five times a day. The only stipulation is to eat a "square meal" every time. The Schwarzbein Square, that is— a balance of quality protein, real carbohydrates, healthy fats and nonstarchy vegetables.

- **Stress Management.** Eight hours of uninterrupted sleep is mandatory on the Schwarzbein Program, as is downtime during the day. I'll show you simple techniques to create both a great night's sleep and daily relaxation.

- **Tapering Off Toxic Chemicals.** Substances such as refined sugars, alcohol, nicotine, artificial sugars, caffeine, and many over-the-counter and prescription drugs have no place in the human body, but some of them are a valuable aid while you transition to a healthy lifestyle. I'll show you how to taper off of toxic chemicals so you won't ever miss them.

- **Smart Exercise.** Moderate exercise is good for you; too much exercise destroys you. Whether you're killing yourself on the couch or on the treadmill, I'll give you a simple routine that will energize and revitalize your body.

- **Hormone Replacement Therapy (HRT).** Not everyone needs HRT, but if your body isn't producing enough of a particular hormone, you will never balance your metabolism, and you will never be truly healthy. I'll show you how to pursue HRT the right way.

Before you move on to the next chapter, take this simple quiz. Did you know that all of the following habits eventually cause fat weight gain or illness? Check the ones that you were not aware of so you understand where your knowledge base is lacking.

❏ Skipping meals
❏ Not eating *enough* carbohydrates, *enough* proteins and/or *enough* fats
❏ Eating *too many* carbohydrates, *too much* protein and/or *too much* fat
❏ Emotional stress
❏ Being too busy
❏ Chronic pain
❏ Not sleeping enough hours or interrupted sleep
❏ Ingesting or using toxic chemicals such as street drugs, tobacco, alcohol, soda, diet soda, refined sugar, caffeine and most medications
❏ Doing too much cardiovascular exercise . . . or not moving at all
❏ Not taking hormone replacement therapy if needed, or taking it incorrectly

Two

The Power of Metabolism: The Science Behind the Schwarzbein Principle

---

Everything you will be learning in my program is based on *known* and *well-grounded* scientific facts found in three major areas of medical study—biochemistry, physiology and endocrinology—and backed up by my clinical experience. For more than 14 years, I have worked with thousands of people to restore balance to their bodies in order to help rid them of many problems, including excess weight, and to reverse or drastically slow the progressive, degenerative diseases of aging. The key is a healthy metabolism.

Metabolism

Wouldn't it be wonderful if the body was so simple that all you had to do is watch how many calories you ate versus how many calories you expended in order to stay thin and healthy? Well, many of you know that it has to be more complicated than that because you may have already been following that advice with mixed results. You know that if "calories in equaled calories out" you would not be searching for new answers as to why you do not have the body composition and overall health you want.

Your metabolism is how your body does what it needs to do: Every day cells in your body are destroyed or damaged by the wear and tear of living, and each day it is the job of your metabolism to regenerate or repair these cells. Your metabolism is also responsible for creating new hormones, enzymes, antibodies, neurotransmitters, other cellular chemicals, energy and energy stores (in the form of fats and glycogen)—and using all it creates to help you perform your daily tasks.

There are two sides to your metabolism: the building side and the using-up side. To be healthy, these two sides must be kept in chemical balance. When you eat well and rest, your body turns into a building machine. When you are not eating, not eating *well* or you are running around doing things, your body switches into using-up mode. Your job is to keep your body functioning efficiently by keeping your metabolism running at its optimum. Because the using-up side is constantly breaking you down, balance can only occur when you give yourself the means to rebuild what you use.

Many people assume the metabolism formula is simple: food becomes energy and activity expends energy. Unfortunately, that is far too simplistic an explanation for what actually goes on in your body. In reality, there are a few more layers. Food, sleep, stress, exercise, toxic chemicals and hormone problems all affect your chemistry.

For instance, food becomes structural and functional chemicals that are used along with energy during the activity of daily life, but processed, damaged foods cannot be used by your body for any legitimate purpose. Furthermore, it is mainly during sleep that your body has the time to rest and catch up on building itself, and if you cut this time short you will not rebuild completely, no matter how healthy your diet. You build more efficiently in the dark than you do in the light, which is why it is important to sleep during the night. You also rebuild slower when it is cold than when it is warm; therefore, you need to sleep more in the winter in order to maintain a balanced metabolism.

The opposite happens with stress and overexercising. When you are under acute or chronic stress, or when you exercise to exhaustion, your body burns itself up more rapidly. This is why fidgety people and heavy exercisers are often thin, but rarely healthy. This is especially true as you get older and your ability to regenerate decreases. The older you are, the harder it is to handle and recover from stress and the more likely cardiovascular exercise will cause irreparable damage to your body.

What about the effects of unnatural or toxic substances? Toxic chemicals like tobacco, alcohol and sugar are temporary boosts that fool your body into thinking it is in better shape than it is. The same is true of caffeine and other stimulants. These chemicals only mask your body's deficiencies; in essence, they rewire your chemistry for a short-term result, but in the end they leave the system disoriented and out of whack. Even worse, these substances don't help the body rebuild, so they cause damage to your metabolism.

A similar phenomenon happens with medicines, both prescription and over-the-counter. Since the dawn of time, the body has used chemicals known as orthomolecules to carry out many of its functions. When you ingest medicine, you displace orthomolecules with foreign substances. This is why, although drugs often help one part of your physiology, most of them cause side effects that are just as bad or worse than what is being treated. You are better off not using any drugs at all, if you can help it.

Do not stop taking your drugs without first consulting your primary care physician. Although most drugs are harmful, you cannot stop using them cold turkey, especially if you have done nothing to fix the underlying problem they were prescribed for in the first place.

Hormones and Their Role in Metabolism

Your hormones are the messengers between the different cells and systems of your body. Hormones relay messages to your cells, which in turn respond by changing their chemical processes. These cells then secrete new hormones that relay messages to other parts of the body. Some of these hormones regulate the rebuilding of your chemicals, while others regulate the use of your chemicals. For you to remain healthy, you need to keep your hormones balanced so they can communicate effectively with each other and with your cells, thereby keeping your metabolism working efficiently.

Hormones are functional chemicals that are made by the cells of your body. In order to produce new hormones, you have to eat food that has the necessary material for your body to make them. Because hormones are mainly made from proteins, cholesterol and essential fats, eating a balanced diet that includes these nutrients is essential for life balance.

Like everything else in your metabolic system, all these hormones are related to and react to one another. In order to maintain an optimal metabolism and remain healthy, your body's hormones need to be kept in balance. If one hormone system is out of balance, they are all out of balance. Thankfully, the opposite also applies. I cannot emphasize this enough: nutrition and lifestyle habits that balance one hormone will help balance all hormones.

However, as you age, your body can lose the ability to make certain hormones. The best known example of this is the loss of estradiol and progesterone hormones when a woman goes through menopause, but most people also lose the ability to regenerate other hormones like DHEA, thyroid and testosterone. That is why an essential part of the Schwarzbein Principle Program is hormone replacement therapy (HRT). Taken at the right time, and in the right way, HRT can be the key to balancing your metabolism and reversing the aging process.

The Aging Process

What is aging? Put simply, it is the breakdown of the building side of your metabolic system—the inability of your body to regenerate itself fast enough to recover from the wear and tear of everyday life.

There are two types of aging: genetic aging and metabolic aging. The first is a product of your heredity; the second is the result of lifestyle choices. When you damage your metabolism through poor choices, you set yourself on an accelerated aging track. But as I said before, the good news is that most of the damage is reversible. That is why building back what you use on a daily basis is essential for health and longevity. It slows the aging process.

You have a predetermined maximum total life span based on the fact that, at a certain point in your life, your cells lose the ability to regenerate. Think of it this way: you only have a certain number of times your cells can turn over (regenerate); if you turn over your cells at a faster rate, you will use yourself up and die sooner. This number of cell turn-overs is determined by your genes and is known as genetic aging. It is a completely normal and inevitable conclusion to life.

You are also born with a predetermined maximum rate of rebuilding. Your genetic ability to rebuild efficiently on a daily basis determines how well you are able to heal from environmental, accidental and self-inflicted damage (poor habits). This rebuilding capacity naturally diminishes as you age. This can be seen in changes in skin, hair, bones, muscles, teeth and nails, slower recovery time from infections, decreased short term memory and physical limitations, such as not being able to run as fast or lift as much weight. Again this is perfectly normal.

You cannot live longer than your preset genetic age, nor can you regenerate faster than your maximum rebuilding rate. However, you can develop more problems, become sicker and die earlier because you are not living up to your body's maximum potential.

Metabolic aging is the type of aging that occurs in relation to daily nutrition and lifestyle habits. You are in control of your metabolic aging because stress, food, toxic chemicals and exercise can either speed up or slow down this process. If you speed up your metabolic aging through poor nutrition and lifestyle choices, you are going to get prematurely ill or die before reaching your maximum life span. This is known as accelerated metabolic or premature aging.

That is what the Schwarzbein Principle Program is all about: making the lifestyle choices that put you in control of your life and slow the aging process. As I said in the last paragraph, nutrition and lifestyle can speed up *or slow down* the effects of aging. Age isn't about the number of years you've been alive, it's about your metabolism's ability to regenerate cells. The less damaged your metabolism, the "younger" your body is—the better you feel, the more energy you have, and the faster your body will burn fat and reach its ideal size and composition.

What About My Excess Fat Weight?

Your health is based on your metabolism functioning optimally, not on your current weight issues. *It is worse to lose weight or to keep weight off by doing all the wrong things than it is to be overweight.* You can be thin and have a damaged metabolism; you can be overweight and have a relatively healthy metabolism. But when your metabolism is completely healthy and you follow this program, you *will* reach the ideal weight and size for your body.

You may be more concerned about your excess fat weight than healing your metabolism because you can see your fat but you can't see your metabolism. And even worse, you know other people can see it, too. Though your feelings are understandable, the issue of your fat weight is secondary to your body's ability to regenerate. You need to eat well to build well, and you need to be healthy to lose weight, not

lose weight to be healthy. That is why my program focuses on healing your metabolism and getting it to work at its optimum level rather than on getting you to lose weight.

When you embrace the fact that your metabolism is more important than your weight, and that a good, healthy life is more important than a trim waist, you will make the necessary changes to your daily habits that will ensure you live longer without disease. And once you have healed your metabolism, you can start burning off your excess fat weight.

Again, this weight loss is a side effect of your improved health, so it may take longer to see the difference in the mirror than it would on that new crash diet, but in the end isn't your health more important? Isn't lifelong fat loss better than another yo-yo diet experience? Does the person who dies skinny really win, even if they die young?

The order of metabolism first, weight loss second is key to changing your life.

Three

The Truth About
Diets and Exercise

In recent decades, our nation's eating habits have swung from a high fat/high protein/low carbohydrate diet to a low fat/low protein/high carbohydrate diet and back to a high fat/high protein/low carbohydrate diet. Along with these eating habits, people have taken numerous diet pills, overexercised and gone through almost every type of torture to try to lose weight. Why do we keep doing this to ourselves when all the data tells us that diets, diet pills and overexercising don't deliver the promised long-term results?

The answer is that Americans are obsessed with being thin, even if it is only short-lived. The first reason for this is fashion. Society has dictated that men and women should look a certain way, and we are all falling for it. How else can we explain the craze of changing eating patterns at the drop of a hat as soon as the latest "scientific" information states that eating a certain way will make you lose the most weight? Whatever happened to balance and moderation in all things?

The second reason for our obsession is health. Many intelligent and conscientious people will change their habits abruptly when any new information comes out regarding habits and health. They will eat vegan, vegetarian, raw foods, food combining, low-fat or

low-carbohydrate diets in the hope that they have found the fountain of youth. They will take up running, spinning, cardiovascular types of yoga or kickboxing because these forms of exercise are being touted as the most healthy. Unfortunately, because these meal and exercise plans cause the body to use up more than rebuild, the person just gets tired, not results. This starts a new search for the latest and greatest program, which usually does the same thing.

How many times in the past twenty years have you heard that eating a low fat, high carbohydrate diet would lower your risk for heart attack and help your weight issues? And that if you were thin you would have less chance of developing high blood pressure, arthritis, diabetes, heart disease and cholesterol problems? Were you at all shocked or dismayed when the same "experts" began recommending that you change your eating habits 180 degrees and eat fewer carbohydrates and more fats to achieve the very same results?!

When a program doesn't work we tend to blame ourselves. We weren't disciplined enough, we didn't follow the program exactly or we aren't good enough. But none of your rationalizations are true. You were disciplined, you did follow the program and you are good enough. It is the popular program that is to blame, not you. If you have a bad program, there will be bad consequences. The actual results will not match the promises.

I cannot say this simple truth enough, so I will say it again: being thin doesn't mean you're healthy. Even if you're losing weight, or near your ideal weight, you may still have an unbalanced metabolism that is sapping your strength, breaking down your body, and leading to degenerative diseases of aging and a shorter life.

The diet industry would have you believe quite the opposite.

They are still promoting weight loss above all else, and they are still advocating the simplistic idea that "calories in" need to be less than "calories used" in order for you to achieve your goal—rapid weight loss. By now you should understand this is flawed thinking that leads to flawed results.

The reason the diet industry is still thriving is that it feels good to lose weight rapidly. Not only will you fit into chic clothes, but you will initially experience an increased sense of well-being and increased energy levels. When your metabolism is in using-up mode, you release anti-inflammatory chemicals, neurotransmitters and endorphins. All of these chemicals make you feel better—less stiff, less depressed and more alive. This all sounds and feels extremely good, but what comes up must come down, and your body will run out of these "feel good" chemicals. When this happens you will be stiffer, you will be more depressed and you will feel more dead than alive.

At this point, most people try something new just to get the original high again. Of course, this is what the industry is banking on. Unfortunately, like almost any drug—and yes, dieting is in many ways a drug—the highs get harder and harder to attain. This is especially true as you get older, because when you are young, your body responds to using up quickly by rebuilding quickly. As you age, it gets harder to rebuild and you no longer have the chemicals needed to make you feel good.

Everyone has a two cents approach to the best way to lose weight quickly, especially when it comes to eating. There are many popular diets that have come and gone throughout the ages, but in the end analysis most are just repeating the failed plans of the past. After all, when your goal is to eat less, there aren't that many ways to change the combination of carbohydrates, fats and proteins that make up the "caloric" part of a diet.

The Six Types of Popular Diets

- **Simple low-calorie diets**—You consume less of everything by counting calories and skipping meals: less protein, fats and carbohydrates.
- **Combined low-calorie diets**—You consume less total food but
  concentrate on eliminating a food group. You can have low-calorie
  combined with low-carbohydrate, low-protein or low-fat intake.
- **Low-fat diets**—You drastically decrease fat intake and eat more
  carbohydrates.
- **Low-carbohydrate diets**—You cut drastically back on carbohydrates and increase fat and protein intake.
- **Food-combining diets**—You eat no carbohydrates, high protein
  and high fat at one meal, and high carbohydrates, no protein and no
  fat at other meals. As long as you don't mix carbohydrates with fats
  and/or proteins, you are food combining.
- **Liquid diets**—You replace solid food with liquid food. Always low
  in total calories.

A Closer Look at Some Popular Diets

No matter what diet program you follow, *if you follow it precisely* you
will initially notice weight loss because the first result of all of them is
that you will pay more attention to how much you eat. The net result,
though, will be that you use up your chemicals faster than you can
rebuild them. You'll lose weight at first, but ultimately you'll crash and
burn. The end result will be that your body becomes so unhealthy that
you can actually start to gain weight *because of your diet!*

Am I saying that all these diets will, in the end, have the same
result? That a low-calorie diet can decrease your health and hurt your
waistline in the same way as a low-fat diet or food-combining diet?

Yes, I am, because in the end they all have the same flawed premise: your body is forced to eat itself up so that you can lose weight.

But with most of these programs the flaws go much deeper.

⊘ Low-Calorie and Calorie-Counting Diets

Premise: The less you eat the better.

Food is probably the most misunderstood lifestyle element in the world today. Many Americans feel, to the detriment of both their bodies and their quality of life, that food is a necessary evil and the less you eat of it the better. These people are skipping meals, starving themselves and feeling guilty about the food they eat.

I'd like to take a moment to remind you of a simple truth: food is essential to life. It is the fuel that runs our bodies and the building material that keeps our muscles and organs strong. Without food, we would die in a matter of weeks. In a world of hunger, it is sad that I have to remind people of the simple fact that food should be enjoyed for the life-giving nourishment, both for the body and the soul, that it provides.

In fact, I go even farther than many diet experts and the well-intentioned family members who tell you to only eat when you are hungry. I completely disagree with this statement. You need to eat well to build well; sometimes hunger has nothing to do with the amount of food you need, especially when your body and mind have been programmed to believe low-level starvation is the way to live.

⊘ Low-Carbohydrate Diets

Premise: Eliminate or severely limit carbohydrates.

Complex carbohydrates are essential to life for a very simple reason: the brain needs them to survive. Here's how they work: Complex carbohydrates are digested into simple sugars. In a special area of your

bloodstream (the portal vein), insulin is released to match the amount of incoming sugar. The insulin communicates to the liver that sugar is waiting to be processed and the liver cells open their doors to let most of the sugar in. The rest of the sugar travels through the liver, out the other end, to the main bloodstream and provides sugar needed for brain and cell function.

Inside the liver cells, the sugar is used for energy, stored as energy or turned into fats. The energy stays in the liver but the fats are released back into the bloodstream where they travel to the other cells of the body. If your body cells need more energy they use this fat as their energy source. If they don't need more energy, they store it as fat. This is why carbohydrates should be a *part* of your healthy diet, not the foundation of your diet.

The brain requires sugar as its main energy source. Since the brain cannot use fat or protein as energy, carbohydrates are essential for good brain health. Therefore, you never want to eliminate or severely limit carbohydrates, not even in the short-term.

Of course, there are bad carbohydrates: they're called refined sugars.

Refined sugars are similar to complex carbohydrates in that both end up as simple sugars. The problem is that refined sugars get broken down and absorbed into the bloodstream (via the portal vein) much quicker and therefore trigger the release of a greater amount of insulin. In response, the liver cells open wider and process simple sugars into fats at a faster rate. In turn, the body's cells open wider and take in more sugar than they need, leaving very little sugar for brain use. This sets up a stress signal in the body. When blood sugar levels start to drop (which they invariably do with refined sugars), the adrenals, the stress glands of your body, release high levels of adrenaline and cortisol (this is the initial rush or "sugar high"). Adrenaline and cortisol cause the proteins of your body to break down and be converted into sugar to fuel the brain—a short-term response with devastating long-term consequences.

⊘ Low-Fat Diets

Premise: Eliminate or drastically reduce fat intake.

Yes, having excess fat around your midsection is bad for your health, but not all fats you eat are bad for you. The healthy fats—monounsaturated (omega-9 fatty acids, olives, avocados, nuts and seeds), polyunsaturated (omega-3 and omega-6 fatty acids, vegetable and fish oils) and saturated (coconut oil, dairy and meat) are essential components of any healthy diet.

Healthy fats are absorbed into the bloodstream (portal vein) or into the lymphatic system, depending on their size. From the portal vein, they go to the liver where they are processed and distributed to the cells of the body. From the lymphatic system, they bypass the liver and go directly into the bloodstream and are delivered unprocessed to the cells of your body. Mono- and polyunsaturated fats are used by all cells mostly as rebuilding materials for structure and function; saturated fats are used by all cells except brain cells mostly for fuel.

Damaged fats like rancid fats, hydrogenated oils or trans-fats (oils found in processed foods such as margarine, breads, donuts, cookies and crackers) are an entirely different story. At the cellular level, they cannot be utilized fully and end up clogging your cells. Or worse, they become incorporated into your cell membranes, replacing healthy fats and affecting the cells' ability to function. Both of these problems cause the cells to die prematurely. In other words, there is no place in the body for damaged fats. They will negatively affect your health and decrease your lifespan.

Fats never become proteins or sugars, so if you only eat fats you will not get the nutrients your body and especially your brain needs. But if you cut them out completely or limit them severely you will be depriving your body of one of its most basic building materials and fuels, and ironically you can become, well . . . fat.

⊘ Food-Combining Diets

Premise: Eat proteins/fats at one meal; eat carbohydrates at the next.

The way you eat your food is as important as how you eat it, but the food combiners have it backward. The healthy way to eat is a balanced diet of all food groups in reasonable portions at all meal times, not separately eating them at different meal times. Food combining is really just another way to use yourself up faster than you can rebuild.

Let's take protein as an example of why an unbalanced diet doesn't work.

Proteins such as beef, poultry, pork, eggs and soy are digested into amino acids (the building blocks of proteins) in the stomach and the small intestine. These amino acids are absorbed into the portal vein where they trigger the release of glucagon, a hormone made in the pancreas that signals the liver that more amino acids need to be processed. If proteins are eaten without any carbohydrates, the glucagon-to-insulin ratio is high, and the signal to the liver is to break down the amino acids and convert them into sugar to fuel the brain. If proteins are eaten with a balanced amount of carbohydrates, the glucagon-to-insulin ratio is low, and the cells of the body will receive the amino acids instead of them being broken down in the liver. The amino acids are now used to rebuild the different proteins that make up the body. Eaten alone, proteins cause you to break down; eaten with the right amount of carbohydrates, they are used to rebuild you. Thus it is very important to always eat a balanced amount of both proteins and carbohydrates—and to eat them at the same time.

Exercise

Another common approach to losing weight is increasing exercise, but again, the health benefits are temporary at best. Ever wonder why

women marathon runners have a higher risk of osteoporosis and low-serotonin problems such as eating disorders and depression? Or why most elite athletes are not long-lived individuals? When you engage in high levels of cardiovascular types of exercise—I call it stimulating exercise because of its effect on the stress hormones in your body—you increase your metabolic rate and use up your body chemicals for energy. This includes not only the normal sources of energy, such as glycogen and fat stores, but also neurotransmitters, enzymes, cellular chemicals or lean body tissue such as bones and muscle. Because you are overtraining, your body needs to "eat" itself up just to keep moving. You do end up losing weight but at the expense of your function and structure, causing damage to your metabolism. Therefore, the more you overexercise to lose weight, the more you will have to exercise to keep it off *because less lean body tissue equates to less fat-burning ability!* Now combine decreasing food intake with increasing exercise and you have a recipe for faster disaster known as accelerated metabolic aging.

Weight-Loss Drugs

Another approach to weight loss is to take prescriptions or over-the-counter drugs that either suppress your appetite (drugs such as phentermine or phen-fen) or increase your metabolic rate (chemicals such as ephedra and ma huang.) The former work on the premise that you will lower your total caloric intake, and therefore they have similar effects as the low-calorie diets. The latter increase the turnover of proteins, fats and carbohydrates and have the same effects as over-exercising. Most of these drugs are now banned because of severe heart complications. Put simply, people died taking them.

Unbelievably, the search continues for the next magic bullet. After all, what is so worrisome about heart disease and death when there is weight to be lost? There are research scientists (paid very well by the

drug companies) hard at work trying to develop new drugs to "help" a person lose weight. I can confidently predict that messing with the body chemistry through newer drugs that affect brain and fat-cell hormone signaling is not going to be any more effective or safer than all the other drugs used to date.

The Results of Unhealthy Weight Loss

The thought behind eliminating fats and/or carbohydrates, eating less food, drinking meals instead of eating them, combining foods in certain ways and taking pills is that anything that helps you lose weight should be good for you. This thought is still accepted because all these programs, in the short term, can cause a decrease in weight, blood pressure and blood sugar levels. This is because they force your body to use up its entire store of energy chemicals, including fat reserves, in a very short amount of time. Things seem to be improving because you are also releasing those "feel good" chemicals, but in reality they are getting worse. Unfortunately, as you are losing "weight" and feeling "better" you are also depleting the essential building material needed for life-sustaining functions.

If you don't believe me, believe your body. How many times have you experienced constipation, headaches, fatigue, dizziness and other symptoms after being on a diet for a longer period of time, especially low-carb and low-fat diets? These are not just temporary conditions; they truly are symptoms of larger problems at work in your body— and they are unequivocally the result of your diet.

The long-term side effects of all unhealthy weight-loss programs include but are not limited to the following:

1. An early death caused by the breakdown of your body systems;
2. Degenerative diseases caused by a lack of the nutrients needed to keep oxidation, inflammation and excessive clotting in check;

3. Autoimmune diseases such as lupus, multiple sclerosis, eczema, ectopic allergies and asthma, Hashimoto's thyroiditis, and rheumatoid arthritis caused by inadvertently stimulating your immune system to attack your own body;

4. Digestive system issues such as unhealthy bacterial or fungal overgrowth and leaky gut syndrome;

5. Fatigue, dizziness, depression, colds, fever, stomachache and other symptoms because you are not getting the nutrients needed for the body to rebuild its function and structure;

6. Headaches, acid reflux, constipation, arthritis pain, sleep disturbances and many other conditions caused by hormone imbalances; and

7. A decrease in lean body tissue and an increase in fat storage, the result of an unhealthy, damaged metabolic system.

You now know why other programs don't work and what kind of damage they can do. It is time to learn why my program does work and what it can do for you.

PART II

The Schwarzbein Program

Four

The Promise of
the Schwarzbein Program:
A Unique Approach to Health

What the Schwarzbein Principle Program will do for you depends on *you*. Your body can regenerate if given the chance. Hopefully by now you are beginning to understand that by following the steps of my program your body will heal itself before burning off its extra fat weight. My program is not simply a weight-loss program, it is a health program. It emphasizes being healthy first, regardless of your weight. If you need to lose fat weight, you will lose it after you heal your metabolism, because when your metabolism is functioning optimally it uses energy to rebuild.

I promise that if you make the necessary changes to give your body what it needs to rebuild and slow how rapidly you use up your chemical resources you will be much healthier in one year. I am not here to lie to you. For those of you who have not fully damaged your metabolism, the effect on your body, your energy and your health will be startling. For those of you with a fully damaged metabolism, you will greatly benefit during the year, but you will not be fully healed. The truth is that it takes years to damage your metabolism and years to repair it.

This may not seem good enough for you, so I ask you to consider

the alternative. What if you keep doing all the wrong things to try to feel better and lose weight quickly? How much more damage can you do in a year? Unfortunately, quite a lot. Your heart health can get worse; your muscles or joints can break down; you can slip into a depressive state because of a depletion of vital chemicals. If you have a degenerative condition, you could lose your ability to live a pain-free life or do the things you love. The simple truth is that if you're not building up your body, you're breaking it down. That means that every day you are living the wrong lifestyle, you are getting less healthy and closer to a premature death.

No matter how damaged your metabolism is at this moment, it can get worse. There is no better time than the present to stop the ongoing destruction and take the time to heal. I am not trying to be an alarmist. I just want you to have all the information you need to make yourself and your health a priority. You are the only one who can do this for yourself, and I encourage you to give yourself the gift of health.

Many people suffer from headaches, heartburn and sleep disturbances without realizing these are symptoms of poor daily habits. If you don't care about the quantity of your life, then make the changes needed to improve the quality of your life. If you are younger than seventy-five years old, you should not and need not have any of the problems listed on the next page. *They are signs of a problem with your metabolism,* and they can completely disappear with improvements in your health habits. If you are older than seventy-five or have a severely damaged metabolism, you can at the very least improve all of these problems. It may just take a little longer to see the results; it takes time to heal.

Each and every one of the following can be completely cured or made much better if you follow the Schwarzbein Principle Program as a way of life.

- Agitation and/or irritability
- Allergies and/or asthma
- Ankle swelling and/or poor circulation
- Anxiety and/or panic
- Chronic pain
- Constipation and/or loose bowel movements
- Depression
- Digestive problems, including intestinal bloating
- Frequent infections and/or poor immune system function
- Headaches not caused by physical trauma
- Irregular heart beats such as palpitations
- Heartburn and other acid reflux problems
- Hypoglycemic symptoms and reactions
- Joint and/or muscle aches and pains
- Low energy levels, including excessive fatigue
- Menopausal symptoms
- Poor memory and concentration
- Premenstrual disorders
- Skin, hair and nail problems
- Sleep issues
- Weakness and/or dizziness
- Weight issues

My program will also help you treat or prevent syndromes such as chronic fatigue syndrome, fibromyalgia and irritable bowel syndrome as well as autoimmune diseases such as Type I diabetes, thyroid problems, lupus, multiple sclerosis, Crohn's disease, ulcerative colitis and rheumatoid arthritis, and the degenerative diseases of aging such as abnormal

cholesterol levels, adrenal gland burnout, some types of cancer, dementia (including but not limited to Alzheimer's), depression, menopause, heart disease (heart attacks, heart arrhythmias, congestive heart failure), high blood pressure disease, morbid obesity (weighing 30 percent or more than your ideal body weight), osteoarthritis, osteoporosis, stroke and Type II diabetes.

An Original Yet Common Sense Approach to Health

I know that you have heard about the five elements of my program from other health-care professionals who advocate eating well, stress management, avoiding toxic chemicals, exercise and hormone replacement therapy. What makes my program different is that it is a step-wise process to healing. These five elements must work together, and in the proper order, for you to truly change your life and your health. Each step of my program is also very specific about the details of changing your lifestyle. For instance, my approach to hormone replacement therapy is based on mimicking normal physiology and avoiding the more commonly prescribed non-bioidentical hormone drugs.

Once again, the five steps of the Schwarzbein Principle Program (SPP) and the purpose of each step are:

Step 1. Healthy nutrition, including taking supplements as needed.

Purpose: By eating enough food from the four food groups and taking supplements as needed, you provide the essential materials and nutrients needed to rebuild your metabolism on a daily basis.

Step 2. Stress management, including getting enough sleep.

Purpose: By managing your stresses better, you slow the using side of your metabolism. By getting enough uninterrupted sleep, you provide your body with the time it needs to rebuild.

Step 3. Tapering off of toxic chemicals or avoiding them completely.

Purpose: By using fewer toxic chemicals or avoiding them completely, you will let your body rebuild more efficiently. However, as you will learn later on, some of these toxic chemicals need to be used during your healing phase as self-medication to enable you to continue your new eating and sleeping habits.

Step 4. Smart exercise.

Purpose: By exercising correctly, you rebuild all proteins, including lean body tissues, and then burn off fat weight.

Step 5. Hormone replacement therapy (HRT), as needed.

Purpose: By taking HRT as needed, you balance your metabolism, thereby slowing the aging process.

In Part III: The Schwarzbein Plans, I will give you specific action plans based on your current metabolism. But first, you need to understand the basic rules for each step of the Schwarzbein Principle Program—and why they are so important to overall health. The next five chapters contain the core elements of my healthy lifestyle program.

As you read these chapters, remember the underlying goal: everything on my program works to balance your hormone systems to heal your metabolism and/or prevent further damage.

Five

Nutrition

> **The Schwarzbein Way:**
> *Never count calories or skip meals. Eat at least three meals and one snack every day. Eat only "square meals" that balance quality proteins, real carbohydrates and healthy fats and supply enough nonstarchy vegetables.*

A key premise behind my program is that you need to eat well to build well and be well. This is accomplished by eating balanced meals and taking the correct supplements, as needed, to provide you with the essential materials and energy to rebuild your metabolism on a daily basis.

The most common mistakes regarding food are the following:

- Not eating enough food or being worried so much about gaining weight that you are always counting your calories;
- Only eating when you are hungry;

- Skipping meals;
- Eliminating a food group;
- Rushing through mealtimes instead of taking the time to chew and digest food properly;
- Drinking instead of eating meals;
- Thinking that taking vitamins and supplements will replace the need for healthy foods; and
- Not taking supplements because you don't like to take pills or think you can get all the nutrients you need from eating well.

Too often, I encounter patients so afraid of food that they are literally starving themselves to death. They have been told again and again that food is the enemy, and they have bought into that so deeply that getting them to eat and not feel guilty can sometimes require psychological therapy—even when the result of their bad habits is that they are underweight and miserable or overweight and miserable. Is this you? Are you afraid of food? If so, you need to know these facts:

- You can gain weight by not eating enough food.
- You can get allergies, asthma, irritable bowel problems, frequent infections and many more problems by avoiding food.
- You can get depressed from not eating well.
- If you are not eating well or eating enough, you are on the accelerated metabolic aging path that will lead to degenerative diseases of aging. You read that right. By counting calories you increase your risk for heart attacks, strokes, diabetes, cancers, osteoporosis, high blood pressure and many more diseases.
- You will shorten your life span if you don't eat well.

If you read the above and still don't care about feeding yourself, you need to see an eating disorder specialist. It is not normal to be afraid of the most important substance on this planet. For the rest of you who are ready to embrace eating well, the following is what you will need to do.

The Ten Nutrition Rules
of the Schwarzbein Principle Program

One: Never skip a meal. When you skip or delay a meal, your body "eats" itself up. You want your body to build itself up, not break itself down. Skipping meals is also a signal for your body to conserve more food as fat the next time you eat. The only way to stop signaling to your body that this is a time of famine and it should conserve more energy as fat is to EAT.

Two: Eat real, unprocessed food. You use food to rebuild your body parts. Foods that you use to rebuild yourself should be real. Real foods are those that you can theoretically pick, gather, milk, fish or hunt. Foods that are highly processed, damaged or filled with toxic chemicals break you down. That is why you need to avoid them as often as possible.

Three: Eat sufficient portions of balanced meals more frequently.
The idea is to eat the right amount of food, not too much and not too little, more frequently throughout the day. You need to eat enough food to keep your body from eating itself up at a given moment but not so much food that it is harder for your body to process it efficiently, leading to increased fat production and storage. You can't win if you eat too much or too little, but it is always better to err on the side of eating more food more often.

Four: Choose a good protein as the main nutrient in your meal.
Your body is made up mostly of proteins, so you will be using proteins as the main material to rebuild with. However, eating too much protein or eating a protein alone triggers you to use up and break down; therefore, you should never eat too much protein or a protein by itself.

Make sure that your protein choice is as fresh as possible and that it is not filled with chemicals, additives, preservatives or hormones. This is a quality protein. Buy organic food as often as possible.

Five: Add real carbohydrates to your meals.

A real carbohydrate is one that can be grown, picked or harvested. Avoid ingesting pesticides by buying organic whole grains, legumes and starchy vegetables as often as possible. It is important to eat the correct amount of carbohydrates. Eating too few carbohydrates breaks you down. Eating too many carbohydrates causes you to overbuild fats, including cholesterol, and to store more fats.

Six: Add some healthy fats to your meal.

It is important to eat enough fat to ensure good brain function, make some of your hormones and keep all your cells happy. The purpose of eating good fats is to rebuild good fats in your body. The key is to eat healthy, nondamaged fats. Avoid all damaged fats found in processed foods. Example of damaged fats are those that are hydrogenated, oxidized or are trans-fats. Do not buy or eat products that contain these types of fats.

Seven: Eat nonstarchy vegetables.

Nonstarchy vegetables are those that do not contain significant amounts of carbohydrates, such as celery, cauliflower, onions, cucumbers, and green and leafy vegetables. This food group adds fiber, vitamins and minerals to your diet, as well as phytochemicals (plant chemicals). These healthy nutrients help your body rebuild tissues and regenerate more quickly. Unfortunately, more and more vegetables contain fewer and fewer nutrients because of nutrient-depleted soil; therefore, I recommend that you supplement with an extremely high-quality multivitamin and mineral.

Eight: Take the time to eat and rotate your foods.

It is important to sit down and take the time to chew your food thoroughly to help you digest properly. You can become allergic to a food if you don't digest it and/or you eat it all the time. Ideally, you don't eat the same food more than once every 2 to 3 days.

Nine: Make sure you drink enough water each day.

Your body is composed of 50 to 60 percent water and it needs to be replaced daily. Drink at least eight full glasses of purified, filtered water a day, more if you are exercising. Do NOT consume high-fructose beverages, artificially sweetened beverages and prepackaged vegetable juices.

Ten: Take supplements as needed.

As you age, your ability to process food and make orthomolecular molecules becomes less efficient. Therefore, supplements are not only beneficial, they become necessary unless you can eat all organic, non-processed, chemical-free foods.

Eat More Food More Often

There is no calorie counting on the Schwarzbein Principle Program. In fact, food is your friend. One of the most dangerous myths in nutrition today is that you should only eat when you are hungry. This is simply not true. One of the tenets of the Schwarzbein Principle Program is something most people will initially find surprising: you should eat at least four, and preferably five, times a day even if you are not hungry. That's right, the motto of this program is that food is your friend, so "gag it down." This is not an endorsement to overeat; it is merely an acknowledgment that many of you—especially the chronic dieters—will at first feel psychologically that you are eating too much on my program. I assure you that you are not.

My reasoning is simple: you have to eat to give your body the energy and materials it needs to rebuild. This is especially true when you are hormonally unbalanced or have a damaged metabolism; you need to heal, so you should be eating *more often* than someone with a healthy metabolism—even if your unhealthy metabolism has led to a weight problem.

Unfortunately, a common symptom of stress or a damaged metabolism is decreased appetite. This causes many people to undereat. You will never heal if you don't eat enough food. You may have to slowly taper up to eating the amount of food that is required for you to heal, but you'll feel better once you do—and once you get over the psychological shock of years of misinformation about diet.

The Schwarzbein Square

Another core tenet of the Schwarzbein Principle Program is the idea of eating "square meals." In this case, I'm referring to the Schwarzbein Square. The rule is simple: each time you eat a meal, you need to consume food from each of the four basic Schwarzbein food groups: quality proteins, real carbohydrates, healthy (undamaged) fats and nonstarchy vegetables. I have designed the Schwarzbein Principle Square to help you visualize how your meals should consist of foods from these four food groups.

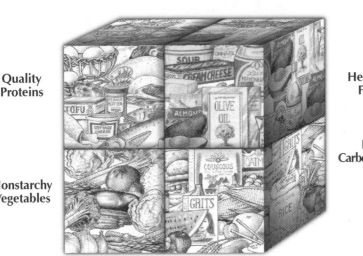

Quality Proteins

Healthy Fats

Real Carbohydrates

Nonstarchy Vegetables

The Schwarzbein Square

How you combine these real foods is as important as eating them. Eating proteins without carbohydrates breaks you down. Eating carbohydrates without proteins builds too much fat. Eating balanced amounts of them together with healthy fats and plenty of nonstarchy vegetables is the key to good health.

In general, to plan a balanced meal divide your plate into one-third slots and place quality proteins, real carbohydrates and nonstarchy vegetables in each slot. Then add healthy fat to some of the portions. For example, a chicken breast, whole grain rice, broccoli and a green salad comprise a quality protein, real carbohydrate and two nonstarchy vegetables. Add a small amount of butter to the rice and use olive oil as part of the salad dressing as your healthy fats. This is a balanced meal. I will go into specifics on exactly what amounts of each food to eat in the plans that conclude this book.

Regarding Digestion

Before I go over the general guidelines for each food group, I want to discuss the importance of digesting and rotating the foods you eat. As important as it is to combine your foods correctly, it is just as important or even more so that the food you eat gets digested properly. If you don't digest your food, you will not be able to absorb your food and, worse yet, you can develop allergies to undigested foods. In both cases, it means that the food you eat cannot be used to rebuild with.

Here are a few simple suggestions to ensure better digestion of your food and to avoid or treat food allergies (see Appendix B for more details):

1) Take the time at mealtimes to sit and eat slowly.
2) Chew your food until it is liquid and then swallow; stop swallowing chunks of food!
3) Drink a full glass of water 1/2 hour before your meal but not during or for up to 30 minutes after your meal. Small sips of water throughout the meal are okay.
4) Take hydrochloric acid and/or digestive enzymes as needed to help you digest your food.
5) It is important to rotate your foods and not eat the same ones over and over again. By eating a variety of foods, you decrease your risk of acquiring a food allergy.

Throughout the next sections look for other helpful hints to help you digest food better.

Proteins

Your body is made up mostly of proteins, so you will be using protein foods as the main material to rebuild with. You can choose quality protein foods such as meats, poultry, fish, eggs, some cheeses and fermented soy options as your protein source. Nuts and nut butters also contain quality protein, but the amount of protein is much lower per serving so they are better reserved for snacks.

———— General Guidelines for Protein Consumption ————

- Eat fresh, organic proteins as much as possible; avoid processed meats that are filled with chemicals, additives, preservatives or hormones.
- Eat only lean meats.
- Eat only nitrate-free meats.
- Eat a variety of different proteins and rotate them so that you do not eat the same proteins daily. This will decrease your risk of developing food allergies.
- Never eat a protein by itself

You are probably eating too much protein if you develop bad breath, get constipated, get stomachaches, cannot sleep well, get irritable, experience heart palpitations, sweat excessively, lose weight too quickly, or experience arthritislike stiffness, inflammation or pain after you start to eat this way.

However, if you have a damaged metabolism you may not feel any symptoms from eating too much protein, so make sure to follow your protein guidelines.

If you feel as if you are not digesting proteins well, you should consider taking betaine hydrochloric acid and/or digestive enzymes. This can be a natural reaction to years of protein deprivation, or you may have a protein allergy. If you think you may have an allergy, follow the

elimination/rotation program found in Appendix B at the end of this book.

PROTEIN FOODS

Eggs, Meat and Poultry

Whenever possible buy hormone-free, antibiotic-free, range-fed meat, poultry and poultry products. Eat lean cuts of meat and more white than dark poultry meat.

Beef*	Pork loin and chops (nitrate- sugar-free bacon
Chicken dark meat*	and ham only occasionally)
Chicken white meat	Quail
Duck and goose*	Squab
Eggs	Turkey dark meat*
Lamb*	Turkey white meat
Pheasant and cornish	Veal
game hens	Wild game

———————
*Limit these on the Healing Plan or if following the lower saturated fat guidelines.

Fish and Shellfish

Fish is an excellent source of protein. Eat fresh wild fish, especially cold water fish high in omega-3 fatty acids, instead of farmed, canned or smoked fish. Stay away from scavenger fish such as catfish, shark, carp and swordfish because they test high for PCBs and other contaminants.

Cheese

As long as you don't have an allergy to cow's milk, you may eat cow's cheese in moderation. If you are allergic to cow's milk, you should be able to tolerate goat, sheep and buffalo cheeses, too. All dairy products should be made from good quality *raw milk that has not been **homogenized and is from cows that have been grass fed. Most imported cheese is raw and made from very high quality milk. Read labels carefully and look for the words fresh milk or milk. You can find raw milk products at *www.realmilk.com* if you are having trouble finding them locally. If you need to eat less saturated fat, you may choose the organic low fat choice of the cheeses found in The Best Cheese to Eat section below.

The Best Cheese to Eat

Cottage cheese	Mozzarella (buffalo	Queso fresco
Feta	and regular)	Ricotta
Goat	Provolone	

Eat Only Occasionally***

Bleu	Cream cheese	Neufchâtel
Brick	Edam	Parmesan
Brie	Fontina	Port de salut
Camembert	Gjetost	Romano
Caraway	Gouda	Roquefort
Cheddar	Gruyère	Swiss
Cheshire	Monterey Jack	Tilsit
Colby	Muenster	

---

* Pasteurization destroys the enzymes found in milk. Therefore, if you eat a pasteurized milk product, you may need to supplement with digestive enzymes to help you digest it. For more information regarding healthy dairy products read Nourishing Traditions by Sally Fallon (New Trends Publishing, 2001).

** Homogenization damages fats.

***Limit these cheeses if you are on the Healing Plan or following the lower saturated fat guidelines.

PROTEIN FOODS THAT CONTAIN CARBOHYDRATES

Count the carbohydrates in these foods as part of your carbohydrate count if you have diabetes or the metabolic syndrome (both are insulin resistant conditions).

Fermented Soy Products

Make sure that you are only eating fermented soy options such as tempeh, natto and miso. Tofu, though not fermented, is okay in small quantities. Other soy food products made from soy protein isolates, textured soy proteins, soy protein powders and soy milk contain natural as well as added chemicals that are harmful to your body. These are not allowed on this program because they are not real foods and cause more harm than good.

Food Item	Serving
Miso (diluted)	¼ cup
Natto	½ cup
Tempeh	½ cup
Tofu	1 cup

Nuts, Nut Butters and Seeds

Most nuts, nut butters and seeds contain quality proteins and healthy fats and real carbohydrates. However, because they don't contain much protein, they are better reserved for snacks than meals. Each serving in the nuts and seeds list found on the next page also contains six grams of carbohydrate, so if you have an insulin resistant condition watch your intake carefully. Eat nuts raw or dry-roasted. All items are raw unless otherwise noted.

Food Item	Serving
Acorns	½ ounce
Almond	1 ounce (23 nuts)
Almond butter	4 tablespoons
Almond paste	½ ounce
Amaranth seed	⅓ ounce
Brazil nuts (butternuts)	1½ ounces
Cashew	¾ ounce
Cashew butter	1½ tablespoons
Chinese chestnuts	½ ounce
Coconut cream	¼ cup
Coconut liquid from coconut	¾ cup
Coconut meat	½ cup, shredded
Coconut milk	½ cup
Cottonseed kernels (roasted)	1 ounce
European chestnuts	½ ounce
Filberts or hazelnuts	1½ ounces
Ginkgo nuts	½ ounce
Hickory nuts	1 ounce
Japanese chestnuts	¾ ounce
Lotus seeds	1½ ounces
Macadamia nuts	1½ ounces
Peanut	1 ounce
Peanut butter	2 tablespoons
Pecans	1 ounce (15 halves)
Pine nuts	1 ounce
Pistachio nuts	1 ounce (47 kernels)
Pumpkin and squash kernels	1 ounce (hulled)
Pumpkin and squash seeds	½ ounce (42 seeds)
Safflower kernels (dried)	½ ounce
Sesame butter (tahini)	1½ tablespoons
Sesame seed kernels (dried)	1 ounce
Sunflower seed butter	1½ tablespoons
Sunflower seed kernels (dried)	¼ cup
Walnuts	2 ounces
Watermelon seed kernels	⅜ cup

PROTEIN FOODS THAT ARE HIGHER IN SATURATED FATS

Eat these foods in moderation if you have a healthy metabolism. Do not eat them at this time if you are following the Healing Plan.

Additive- and Nitrate-Free Sausages

Many communities have at least one old-fashioned butcher shop that still makes homemade sausages. Do not eat them if they are not additive- and nitrate-free. Avoid eating sausages completely on the Healing Plan or if you are following the lower saturated fat guidelines. The rest of you should limit your intake to one to two servings a week at the most or not at all. Never eat processed sausage or lunch meats because they contain nitrates (that increase your risk for developing cancer) and/or added sugar.

Berliner	Duck sausage	Liver sausage
Bockwurst	Frankfurter	Liverwurst
Bratwurst	Italian sausage	Polish sausage
Braunschweiger	Kielbasa	Pork and beef sausage
(liverwurst)	Knackwurst	Pork sausage
Chicken sausage	Liver cheese	Turkey sausage
Chorizo		

Pâté

Limit pâté to one to two servings a week. However, eat less if you are also consuming other proteins high in saturated fats. Do not eat if you are on the Healing Plan or are following the lower saturated fat guidelines.

Protein Powders

In general, it is better to eat real food than to add protein powders. However, if you are in a bind or have severe food allergies, it is better to use protein powders than not to eat any protein at all. However, do not use soy protein powders. The best powders to use are made from whey or rice proteins.

Carbohydrates

Your body uses carbohydrates mostly for energy; therefore eating too few or too many carbohydrates is equally damaging. Carbohydrates that are acceptable on this program are starchy vegetables, legumes, whole grains and cereals, some types of milk products, fruits and vegetable juices. Nonacceptable carbohydrates are refined grains and cereals, sugary foods, fruit juices and alcohol. (There are minor exceptions to this in the SPP plans.)

General Carbohydrate Guidelines

- Eat real carbohydrates as much as possible—man-made carbohydrates usually contain a lot of refined sugars and other chemicals. Read labels carefully. A real carbohydrate is one that can be grown, picked or harvested.
- Eat carbohydrates to match your current metabolism and activity level.
- Never eat a carbohydrate by itself.
- Avoid pesticides and genetically modified foods by buying organic fruits, whole grains, legumes and starchy vegetables as much as possible.
- Buy sprouted grains and legumes or soak them yourself overnight to predigest them. This improves your ability to digest and absorb them and helps to decrease the risk of developing food allergies.

ACCEPTABLE CARBOHYDRATES

Starchy Vegetables

All items are cooked unless otherwise noted. Each of the following serving sizes contains approximately 15 grams of carbohydrate.

Food Item	Serving
Acorn squash	½ cup
Artichokes	1 artichoke
Beets	1 cup
Burdock root (raw)	½ root
Butternut squash	⅔ cup
Carrots	1 cup
Corn	½ cup
Green peas	½ cup
Jerusalem artichokes	½ cup
Jicama	⅔ cup
Leeks	1 cup
Lima beans	½ cup
Lotus root	½ cup
Okra	1 cup
Parsnip	⅔ cup
Potato (baked)	½ medium
Pumpkin	1 cup
Rutabaga (raw)	¼ large
Sweet potato or yam	½ medium
Turnip	½ cup

Legumes

Legumes need to be sprouted or soaked overnight before they are eaten to ensure their proper digestion and absorption. Or better yet, buy biodynamically grown legumes if you are too busy to worry about this (check out the food store at www.westonaprice.com for sources).

All items are cooked unless otherwise noted. Each of the following serving sizes contains approximately 15 grams of carbohydrate.

Food Item	Serving
Adzuki beans	¼ cup
Black beans	⅓ cup
Broadbeans (fava beans)	½ cup
Chickpeas (garbanzo, Bengal)	⅓ cup
Cowpeas (black-eyed peas)	½ cup
Cranberry (Roman) beans	⅓ cup
French beans	⅓ cup
Garbanzo beans	⅓ cup
Great Northern beans	⅓ cup
Hominy	½ cup
Hyacinth beans	⅓ cup
Kidney beans	⅓ cup
Lentils	⅓ cup
Lupins	1 cup
Moth beans	⅓ cup
Mung beans	⅓ cup
Mungo beans (dry)	½ cup
Navy beans	⅓ cup
Pigeon peas	⅓ cup
Pink beans	⅓ cup
Pinto beans	⅓ cup
Split peas	⅓ cup
White beans	⅓ cup
Yellow beans	⅓ cup

Whole Grains and Cereals

Buy whole grains that are packaged and not in bins to avoid cross-contamination and because they are fresher. Avoid genetically modified grains because the foreign proteins can cause intestinal irritation and/or allergies. Avoid eating processed grains. Never eat grains that are "flavored" or that have additives such as imitation bacon bits.

Each of the following serving sizes contains approximately 15 grams of carbohydrate.

Food Item (cooked unless noted)	Serving
Barley*	⅓ cup
Brown rice	⅓ cup
Buckwheat (whole-grain)	⅓ cup
Buckwheat groats (kasha)	⅓ cup
Bulgur (tabouli)*	⅓ cup
Cold cereal*+	read label
Corn bran (crude)	¼ cup
Corn grits, white or yellow	½ cup
Couscous farina*	⅓ cup
Millet	⅓ cup
Oats**	⅔ cup
Polenta	⅓ cup
Popcorn (air-popped)	2½ cups
Quinoa	⅓ cup
Rye*	¼ cup
Semolina (whole-grain, dry)*	2 tablespoons
Triticale (dry)*	2½ tablespoons
Wheat (whole-grain, dry)*	1½ tablespoons
Wheat bran (crude, dry)*	½ cup
Wheat germ (crude, dry)*	⅓ cup
Wild rice	½ cup

*Contain gluten—avoid if you have a gluten allergy or are following the Healing Plan.

** If you are allergic to gluten but do not have full-blown celiac disease, you may still be able to tolerate oats. Make sure you buy them packaged, not from bins, from a mill that avoids cross-contamination with other grains. Read package labels.

+ Made from organic grains and without hydrogenated fats or high amounts of added sugar.

Whole Grains—Flours and Meals

It is better to eat the whole grain than to use flours and meals. However, small amounts will not break this program.

Each of the following serving sizes contains approximately 15 grams of carbohydrate. All items are dry.

Food Item	Serving
Almond meal	½ cup
Amaranth flour	2 tablespoons
Arrowroot flour	2 tablespoons
Brown rice flour	2 tablespoons
Buckwheat flour (whole-grain)	3½ tablespoons
Corn flour (whole-grain)	2½ tablespoons
Cornmeal	2 tablespoons
Cottonseed flour	1½ ounces
Oat bran flour*	⅔ cup
Peanut flour	⅔ cup
Pecan flour	¾ cup
Potato flour	1½ tablespoons
Rye flour*	3 tablespoons
Semolina flour (whole grain)*	2 tablespoons
Sesame flour	2½ tablespoons
Soy flour	½ cup
Sunflower seed flour	¾ cup
Triticale flour*	2½ tablespoons
Whole-wheat flour*	3 tablespoons

*Contain gluten—avoid if you have a gluten allergy or are following the Healing Plan.

Breads and Tortilla Exceptions

In general, I don't want you to consume man-made carbohydrates. The following selections are the exception. Please read the disclaimers that accompany them carefully. Each serving contains approximately 15 grams of carbohydrates.

Food Item	Serving
Corn tortilla, without additives or preservatives	1 medium
Homemade or bakery sprouted whole grain breads, without additives, preservatives, damaged fats or high amounts of sugar*	1/2 to 1 slice
Sourdough bread, made with whole ingredients only**	1/2 slice

---

* contain gluten

** If you have a gluten intolerance, not full-blown celiac disease, you may be able to tolerate sourdough bread because the souring process can predigest some of the gluten. However, do not try eating it until you have been gluten free for at least six months. If you reintroduce it and react poorly, stop eating it for now and try again in another six months or make your own sourdough bread. (refer to www.westonaprice.org/foodfeatures/ourdailybread.html for a good recipe.). If you still react after a year this will probably never work for you.

Yogurt

Though yogurts contain protein, fats and carbohydrates, they are still considered a carbohydrate food. You can count the protein and fat in them towards your personal requirements. Refer to the Plans at the back of this book. Only eat organic yogurt. Eat yogurts made from goat, sheep or buffalo milk if you have a dairy (casein) allergy and read the labels to make sure casein was not added to them. There are reduced saturated fat organic yogurts. Eat these if you are following the Healing Plan or the lower saturated fat guidelines.

Each of the following serving sizes contains approximately 15 grams of carbohydrate.

Food Item	Serving
Organic plain whole milk, cow	1 cup
Organic plain whole milk, goat	1 cup
Organic plain whole milk, Indian buffalo	1 cup
Organic plain whole milk, sheep	1 cup

FRUITS

Fruits are high in simple sugar. However, they also contain vitamins, minerals and fiber, so they are an acceptable form of carbohydrate in moderation.

The "Fruit Servings" lists on the next two pages divide the different fruits by sugar load—lowest, intermediate, highest. The best fruit choices are the ones with the lowest sugar load. However, if you have a healthy metabolism, you can eat other fruits as described in the Maintenance Plan section.

Eat fruits in their natural state and make sure they are organic and "spray-free." Do not drink fruit juices, eat fruit cocktail or fruits canned in syrup because they contain too much sugar. (If you have a healthy metabolism, it is okay to drink small amounts of fruit juices—see the Maintenance Plan.)

Fruit Serving by Sugar Load

Each portion size is equal to 15 grams of carbohydrate.

Lowest Sugar Load*

Blackberries	¾ cup
Blueberries	½ cup

Fruit Serving by Sugar Load (cont'd)

Boysenberries	¾ cup
Grapefruit	½ medium or ½ cup
Raspberries	1 cup
Strawberries	1¼ cups

Intermediate Sugar Load

Apple	1 small
Applesauce (unsweetened)	½ cup
Apricots	2 medium
Apricot halves	4 halves
Cantaloupe	1¼ cups
Cherries	12 cherries
Honeydew	⅛ medium
Kiwi	1 large
Mango	½ small
Nectarine	1 small
Orange	1 small
Papaya	1 cup
Peach	1 medium
Pear	½ large
Pineapple (raw)	¾ cup
Plums	2 medium

————————

These are the only fruits allowed on the Healing Plan.

Fruit Serving by Sugar Load (cont'd)

Highest Sugar Load

Banana	½ small
Dates	2 medium
Figs	2 medium
Grapes	15 small
Prunes	3 medium
Raisins	2 tablespoons
Watermelon	1¼ cups

Combined Fruit List

Each of the following serving sizes contains approximately 15 grams of carbohydrate. All fruits are raw, except when noted.

Food Item	Serving
Acerola (West Indian cherry)	15 fruits
Apple	1 small
Apples (dried)	3 rings
Applesauce (unsweetened)	½ cup
Apricots	2 medium
Apricots (dried)	7 halves
Avocado (California)	1 avocado
Avocado (Florida)	½ avocado
Banana	½ small
Bananas (dehydrated)	1 tablespoon
Blackberries	¾ cup
Blueberries	½ cup
Boysenberries	¾ cup
Breadfruit	⅛ small
Carambola (starfruit)	1½ cups (sliced)
Cherimoya (custard apple)	2 ounces

Combined Fruit List (cont'd)

Food Item	Serving
Cherries	12 cherries
Crabapple	½ cup (sliced)
Cranberries (unsweetened)	1 cup, whole
Currants (European, fresh)	1 cup
Currants (red or white)	1 cup
Currants (Zante, dried)	2 tablespoons
Dates	2 medium
Elderberries	½ cup
Figs	2 medium
Figs (dried)	1 medium
Gooseberries	1 cup
Grapefruit	½ medium or ½ cup
Grapes (American)	15 grapes
Grapes (European)	7 grapes
Groundcherries (cape gooseberries)	1 cup
Guavas (common)	1½ guavas
Guavas (strawberry)	15 guavas
Jackfruit	2 ounces
Java-plum (Jambolan)	¾ cup
Jujube	¼ cup
Jujube (dried)	1 tablespoon
Kiwi fruit (Chinese gooseberries)	1 large
Kumquats	5 kumquats
Lemons	3 medium
Limes	2 medium
Litchis	7 fruits
Litchis (dried)	2 tablespoons
Loganberries	¾ cup
Longans	31 fruits
Longans (dried)	2 tablespoons

Combined Fruit List (cont'd)

Food Item	Serving
Loquats	5 large
Mammey-apple	1 medium
Mango	½ small
Melon (cantaloupe)	1¼ cups (cubes)
Melon (casaba)	1½ cups (cubes)
Melon (honeydew)	⅛ medium
Mulberries	1 cup
Nectarine	1 small
Orange	1 small
Papaya	1 cup
Passion fruit (granadilla)	3 fruits
Peach	1 medium
Peaches (dried)	2 halves
Pear	½ large
Pears (dried)	1 half
Persimmon (Japanese)	½ medium
Persimmon (Japanese, dried)	½ medium
Persimmons (native)	2 medium
Pineapple	¾ cup
Plantains (cooked)	⅓ cup
Plums	2 medium
Pomegranates (Chinese apple)	½ fruit
Pomelo	¾ cup
Prickly pears	1½ medium
Prunes	3 medium
Quince	1 medium
Raisins (dark/golden seedless)	2 tablespoons
Raspberries	1 cup
Rhubarb	7 stalks
Rose-apples	2 medium

Combined Fruit List (cont'd)

Food Item	Serving
Sapotes (marmalade plum)	½ medium
Soursop (guanabana)	½ cup
Strawberries	1¼ cups
Sugar-apple (sweetsop)	½ fruit
Sun-dried tomatoes	⅙ ounce
Tamarinds	15 fruits
Tangerines	2 small
Tomatillo	1 large
Tomato (green and red)	1 medium
Watermelon	1¼ cups

Vegetable Juices

The following are a few vegetable juices that are acceptable to drink if they are not filled with additives, preservatives, high amounts of salt or added sugar. The best juices are the ones you make with fresh ingredients at home.

Note: Do not drink these if you have an insulin resistant condition.

Food Item	Serving
Carrot	3 fluid ounces
Tomato	6 fluid ounces
Vegetable	6 fluid ounces

CARBOHYDRATES TO EAT OCCASIONALLY

Man-Made Carbohydrate Options

The goal is to eliminate all man-made carbohydrates, especially on the Healing Plan. However, if you do eat them, some man-made carbohydrates are better than others. Each of these man-made carbohydrate selections contains 15 grams of carbohydrate.

Please read labels and avoid all man-made carbohydrates that have partially hydrogenated and/or hydrogenated fats as well as added sugar.

Breads

Fresh-baked bread is preferable because it contains no additives.

Food Item	Serving
Bread crumbs (whole wheat)*	1½ tablespoons
Cracked-wheat bread*	1 slice
Cracker meal*	1½ tablespoons
French bread*	½ to 1 slice
Irish soda bread*	½ to 1 slice
Italian bread*	½ to 1 slice
Low-carbohydrate bread**	2 slices
Oat bran bread*	1 slice
Oatmeal bread*	1 slice
Pumpernickel bread*	1 regular slice
Rice bran bread	1 slice
Rye bread*	1 large slice
Wheat bran bread*	1 slice
Wheat germ bread*	1 slice
Wheatberry*	1 slice
Whole-grain dinner roll*	1 roll
Whole-grain English muffins*	½ muffin
Whole-grain hamburger/hot dog bun*	½ slice
Whole-grain pita*	1 small pita
Whole-grain raisin bread*	1 slice
Whole-grain, 7-grain bread *	1 slice

Contain gluten—avoid if you have a gluten allergy or are following the Healing Plan.
**This is any bread with 7½ grams of carbohydrate or less.*

Crackers

Most crackers contain many additives, including hydrogenated fats. Look for crackers that are low-carbohydrate, whole-grain and do not contain any type of hydrogenated fats. Each selection below contains 15 grams of carbohydrate.

Food Item	Serving
Rice crackers	4 crackers
Rusk toast*	1½ ounces
Rye crispbread*	2 crackers
Rye wafers (Wasa) *†	2 crackers
Wheat crackers (Ak-Mak) *†	4 crackers
Wheat Euphrates *†	5 crackers
Wheat melba toast*	3 toasts
Whole-wheat matzo*	½ (6"x 4") matzo

*Contains gluten.
†Best choices if you do not have a gluten allergy and are on the Maintenance Plan.

Refined Grains and Cereals

Do not eat puffed grains, including rice cakes. The high heat used to process them is very damaging and creates free radicals.

Cream of rice   Cream of wheat*   White rice

*Contains gluten.

OTHER MAN-MADE CARBOHYDRATE PRODUCTS

If you have a healthy metabolism and are eating well, managing your stresses, getting enough sleep and doing moderate amounts of the right types of exercise, small amounts of these foods occasionally will not break your program. However, as much as possible try eating real carbohydrates that are grown or picked. Read labels carefully and make sure that you are not eating man-made carbohydrates that have hydrogenated fats or lots of added sugar.

Refined Breads

These breads are usually made with refined white flour. Only eat these occasionally and only if you are following the Maintenance Plan and you do not have a gluten allergy. I cannot emphasize enough that you need to make sure that they are not filled with sugar and hydrogenated fats.

Bagels	Dinner rolls	English muffins
Bread sticks	Egg bread	Flour tortilla

Bakery Goods

If you have a healthy metabolism, you may occasionally have the following foods if they are made from organic grains and flours and they are not filled with sugar and hydrogenated fats. This means that you probably will be making your own.

Banana bread*	Croutons*	Popovers*
Biscuits*	Crumpets*	Puff pastry*
Bread stuffing*	Muffins*	Scones*
Corn cakes	Pancakes*	Waffles*
Cornbread	Phyllo dough*	Wonton wrappers*
Cornbread stuffing	Pie crust*	
Croissants*	Pizza dough*	

Contain gluten unless made with gluten free flours.

Pretzels and Chips

Only eat baked chips and those without damaged fats. Eat whole-wheat pretzels without hydrogenated fats only.

Corn chips	Pretzels*	Tortilla chips
Potato chips	Taro chips	

Contain gluten.

Pizza and Pasta

In general, pasta is not a good source of carbohydrates because it is devoid of anything but the flour. If you don't have an allergy to wheat or gluten, you may have small amounts of organic whole-grain pastas that do not contain hydrogenated oils as long as you have a healthy metabolism. Read labels. Look for wheat-free, gluten-free pasta alternatives usually made from beans if you are a pasta-lover and want to eat pasta more frequently. Do not eat pasta made from soy bean products. If you have a healthy metabolism, you can eat whole grain, thin crust pizza with sugarless sauce on occasion.

Acceptable Desserts

In general, it is better to avoid sugary foods as much as possible. However, if you have a healthy metabolism, small amounts of organic desserts made with whole food and flour products will not make or break your program. Make sure that they are not filled with hydrogenated fats. Most likely you will need to make these at home because you won't be able to find prepared products that qualify.

Cakes*	Fruit butters	Jams, jellies, marmalade and preserves
Cheesecake*	Ice cream	Pies
Cookies*	(whole fat only)	

*Usually contain gluten.

Sugars

Small amouts of honey or molasses will not break your program if you have a healthy metabolism. The only other sweeteners I endorse are Stevia and small amounts of xylitol.

Fats

Do not be afraid to eat real foods that contain healthy fats, including cholesterol. Not all fats are harmful; in fact, healthy fats are essential for optimum health because they give you energy and are used to rebuild your body. Eating healthy fats will keep you happier and healthier longer by allowing your body to maintain hormone balance and slowing down accelerated aging. Healthy fats are required for normal cell function, a healthy immune system, for the absorption of fat-soluble vitamins, as an energy source, and to slow the absorption of carbohydrates and proteins. This will keep you satiated and satisfied so that you don't overeat other foods.

Healthy fats include naturally occurring saturated fats and non-damaged mono- and polyunsaturated oils. When you are looking for non-damaged oils, check the label for cold-pressed, pure-pressed or expeller-pressed oils and that they are packaged in opaque containers to keep them fresh longer.

Though saturated fats have been getting a bad rap, they are not bad for you as long as they are natural and you can process them for energy. These are the fats found in animal and tropical oils. Man-made saturated fats such as margarine and shortening, made from hydrogenating polyunsaturated vegetable oils, are very damaging. You will not be eating any of these on this program.

On the other hand non-damaged polyunsaturated oils are your body's only source for the essential fatty acids known as the omega-3 and omega-6 fatty acids. A good balance between these two types of fats is when you consume no more than 3 to 1 omega-6 to omega-3 fatty acids. This means that you need to eat at least one gram of omega-3 fatty acids for every three grams of omega-6 fatty acids.

Although in theory you do not have to count or measure your fat intake, strive for moderation. You should not overeat fats, just like you should not overeat carbohydrates or proteins. This is not a high-fat or low-fat eating plan; it is a balanced eating plan.

A general rule regarding fat intake is that the total fat you eat should not exceed 50 to 60% of your total daily caloric intake, but you will need to eat less than this if you have a severely damaged metabolism. Most of the fat you eat should be saturated and monounsaturated. Only a small amount should be polyunsaturated.

——— **General Guidelines for Fat Consumption** ———

* Eat healthy, not damaged, fats.
* Eat fresh fats and keep fats refrigerated.
* Use natural saturated fats or monounsaturated oils for cooking.
* Keep monounsaturated and polyunsaturated oils in opaque, airtight containers.
* Read labels to avoid buying fats with added chemicals.
* Cook fatty meats at low, even temperatures to avoid damaging fats.
* Cook your eggs at low, even temperatures. (Egg yolks have essential fatty acids and other polyunsaturated fats that can be damaged at high heat.)

The key to the Schwarzbein Principle Program is to avoid damaged fats, such as fats found in processed foods. Examples of damaged fats are those that are hydrogenated, oxidized, rancid or are trans-fats. Do not buy or eat products that contain these types of fats.

The Don'ts of Fats

* Do not cook with polyunsaturated oils.
* Do not cook with butter at high temperatures. Butter contains polyunsaturated oils and can be damaged with high heat. You can use natural saturated or monounsaturated fats to cook with because they are more resistant to damage from high temperatures.
* Do not use most low-fat or nonfat products as the fat is usually replaced with sugars and/or artificial chemicals.
* Do not eat a fat *food* by itself.

ACCEPTABLE FATS

Fats and Oils

It is important to know that all fats and oils are a combination of saturated, mono and polyunsaturated fatty acids. The lists below have the fats listed in the category that describes their fat content best.

In general, use mostly natural saturated fats and pure-pressed, cold-pressed or expeller-pressed monounsaturated oils; only use pure-pressed, cold-pressed or expeller-pressed polyunsaturated oils in small amounts.

Saturated	Monounsaturated	Polyunsaturated
Butter*	Almond oil	Corn oil
Chicken fat*	Avocado oil	Cottonseed oil
Coconut oil**	Canola oil****	Essential fatty acids
Cream***	Duck fat**	(borage, flaxseed,
Palm and palm	Goose fat**	primrose)
kernel**	High oleic	Ghee (clarified butter)
Tallow	safflower and	Safflower oil
Turkey fat	sunflower oils*****	Salmon oil
	Olive oil	Sesame oil
	Peanut oil******	Sunflower oil
		Wheat germ oil

---

* Butter and chicken fat contain quite a bit of polyunsaturated oils so they should not be used to cook with at high heat.

** Coconut and other tropical oils can be used freely when cooking and baking because of their high saturated and monounsaturated fat content. The same goes for duck and goose fat.

*** Use only organic heavy whipping cream without any added chemicals.

**** Canola oil is mostly a monounsaturated fat and, though most of the harmful erucic acid has been bred out of most commercial forms of Canola oil, it still presents a problem because, among other reasons, during the process of extracting it the omega-3 fatty acids are transformed into trans-fats. If you are going to still use this oil, use it in small amounts and make sure that you eat enough saturated fats in your diet to help offset some of its potential risks.

***** High oleic safflower and sunflower oils, produced from hybrid plants, are similar to olive oil and can be used, as can olive oil, to cook with as long as they are cold-pressed.

****** Peanut oil should be used sparingly to cook with because it contains a fair amount of omega-6 fatty acids.

Food Sources of Omega-3 Fatty Acids

Consume at least two to three grams of omega-3 fats per day.

Food	Serving Size	Omega-3 Content (gms)
FISH		
Fatty fish: wild salmon, sardines, mackerel, bluefin or albacore tuna, bluefish	3½ ounces	1.0–2.5
Medium-fat fish: trout, rockfish, oysters, mussels	3½ ounces	0.5–0.8
Low-fat fish: halibut, crab, cod, flounder, scallops, lobster, clams, swordfish, sole, orange roughy, shrimp	3½ ounces	0.1–0.4
MEAT		
Lamb	3½ ounces	0.5
Meat, poultry	3½ ounces	0.2
Dairy products	1 ounce cheese	0.1
NUTS AND SEEDS		
Walnuts	2 tablespoons	1.0
Chia seeds	2 tablespoons	1.1
OILS		
Flax oil	1 tablespoon	6.6
Flax meal	1 tablespoon	1.6
Canola oil	1 tablespoon	1.6
LEGUMES AND TOFU		
Soybeans, cooked	1 cup	1.1
Tofu, firm	½ cup	0.7
VEGETABLES		
Purslane	3½ ounces	0.4
Broccoli, kale, leafy greens	½ cup	0.1
Peas	½ cup	0.1

Food Sources of Omega-6 Fatty Acids

You should eat no more than approximately *three times* the amount of omega-6 fats as omega-3 fats.

Food	Serving Size	Omega-6 Content (gms)
PLANT FOODS		
Fats and Oils		
Safflower oil	1 tablespoon	10.0
Sunflower oil	1 tablespoon	9.0
Corn oil	1 tablespoon	8.0
Mayonnaise	1 tablespoon	5.0
Peanut oil	1 tablespoon	4.5
Olive oil	1 tablespoon	1.2
Nuts and Seeds		
Seeds (sesame, pumpkin, sunflower)	¼ cup	9.0
Nuts (peanuts, walnuts, Brazil and pine nuts)	1 ounce	4.0
Nuts (almonds, cashews, pecans, hazelnuts)	1 ounce	2.0
Legumes/Whole Grains		
Tofu, firm	½ cup	5.4
Soybeans (cooked from dry)	½ cup	3.6
Tofu, medium	½ cup	3.5
Wheat germ	2 tablespoons	1.0
Grains (wheat, rice, oats, etc.)	½ cup cooked	0.5
Legumes	½ cup	0.2
Vegetables and Fruits		
Avocado	1 whole	3.5
Vegetables and fruits	½ cup or 1 medium fruit	0.05
ANIMAL FOODS		
Meat, Poultry and Fish		
Poultry (light and dark meat)	3½ ounces	2.0
Pork (lean)	3½ ounces	0.7
Beef (lean)	3½ ounces	0.3
Fish (high-fat varieties)	3½ ounces	0.2
Fish (low-fat varieties)	3½ ounces	0.1

Saturated Fats

Though saturated fats in theory are not bad for you, they will cause problems if you cannot burn them for energy. It is easier to metabolize short chain saturated fats found in butter and coconut oil than it is to metabolize the longer chain saturated fats found in margarine, shortening and animal fats. Here is a list of foods to avoid that contain high amounts of long chain saturated fats and ones to use in their place. Foods with less than three grams of longer chain saturated fat per serving are considered to be low saturated fat foods. You will be following a low saturated meal plan if you have a damaged metabolism or you need to lose excess fat weight.

Lower Saturated Fat Guidelines

DAIRY:

Food Recommendations:

As long as you eat raw organic cheeses and yogurts made from whole fat milk products, you may still consume normal amounts of them when following the lower saturated fat guidelines. You can also eat their reduced fat counterparts if they are organic.

MEATS:

Foods to Avoid:

* Red meat
* Sausage, ham, bacon, dark chicken meat and skin, dark turkey meat and skin, duck, goose, ribs, highly marbled meats and prime grades of meat

Low Saturated Fat Guidelines (cont'd)

Food Recommendations:

• Fish and poultry (only white meat)
• Lean cuts of pork and lamb
• Ground sirloin in place of ground beef, but limit to once or twice a week

FATS, OILS AND FOODS WITH FAT:
Foods to Avoid:

• Lard, cream sauces and dressings
• Margarine and shortening

Food Recommendations:

• Extra virgin olive oil
• Avocado, olives, nuts and organic nut butters
• Moderate amounts of raw organic butter, coconut oil and palm oil
• Small amounts of duck and goose fat

Nonstarchy Vegetables

Nonstarchy vegetables are a source of fiber, vitamins and minerals. The fiber slows the digestion and absorption of your carbohydrates, proteins and fats. This helps balance your hormones and at the same time allows only a small amount of food to enter your bloodstream at any given moment. This is important because your body is able to process food better in smaller quantities.

Fiber also helps add bulk to your bowel movements and is what good colon bacteria use as food to thrive. This helps keep your colon healthy and happy.

The vitamins and minerals found in nonstarchy vegetables are used as coenzymes, which are chemicals that speed up biochemical reactions. This helps you regenerate more efficiently.

——— General Nonstarchy Vegetables Guidelines ———

• Consider any vegetable that contains five grams or less of carbohydrate per half-cup serving to be a nonstarchy vegetable.

• Eat at least five servings of nonstarchy vegetables a day and include at least one serving with each meal, including breakfast.

• Eat organically grown vegetables as often as possible to avoid pesticides.

• Vary your choices for optimum health and to decrease the chance of becoming allergic to them.

• You may eat frozen vegetables as long as there are no added preservatives or sugars. Watch out for hidden salt in frozen vegetables if you have water-retention problems such as ankle swelling and bloating.

• Carrots and tomatoes are considered both starchy and nonstarchy vegetables. When you eat them raw, consider them nonstarchy. When you cook them, consider them starchy. (Cooking breaks down their fiber content.)

ACCEPTABLE VEGETABLES

Nonstarchy Vegetables

Amaranth leaves
Arrowhead
Arugula
Asparagus
Balsam-pear
Bamboo shoots
Bean sprouts
Beet greens
Bell peppers
  (red, green, yellow)
Borage
Broadbeans
Broccoli
Brussels sprouts
Butterbur (fuki)
Cabbage
Cardoon
Carrots (raw)
Cassava
Cauliflower
Celeriac
Celery
Celtuce
Chayote fruit
Chicory (witloof)
Chicory greens
Chives

Chrysanthemum
  (garland)
Collard greens
Coriander
Cowpeas (leafy tips)
Cucumber
Dandelion greens
Dock
Eggplant
Endive
Eppaw
Fennel
Gardencress
Garlic
Ginger root
Gourd
Green beans
Hearts of palm
Horseradish-tree,
  leafy tips/pods
Jalapeño peppers
Jew's ear (pepeao)
Jute potherb
Kale
Kohlrabi
Lamb's quarter
Lettuce

Mushrooms
Mustard greens
Nopales
Onions
Parsley
Peppers (sweet green,
  red and yellow)
Pokeberry shoots
Pumpkin flowers/
  leaves
Purslane
Radicchio
Radishes
Salsify
Scallop squash
Sesbania flower
Shallots
Snap beans
Snow peas
Spaghetti squash
Spinach
Summer squash
  (crookneck,
  scallop,
  straight neck,
  zucchini)
Sweet potato leaves

Nonstarchy Vegetables (cont'd)

Swiss chard

Taro (leaves or
  shoots)

Tomatoes (raw)

Tree fern

Turnip greens

Watercress

Waxgourd (Chinese
  preserving melon)

Herbs and Spices

Spices and herbs do not contain sugar. Use them freely.

Healthy Condiments

Balsamic and other vinegars

Garlic cloves

Homemade sauces

Low-sodium tamari soy sauce*

Natural mustard

Olives

Peanut sauce (made without sugar)

Salsa (made without sugar)

*May contain gluten.

Beverages

It is important to drink enough fluids throughout the day. Being dehydrated affects you in many ways. You can mistake thirst for hunger, have a harder time burning off fat weight, increase your risk for ulcers and arthritis, decrease your energy levels, decrease your ability to think and increase your risk for cancers. Do something easy and good for yourself. Keep well hydrated.

What to Drink

Water

This is the best choice. Your body is comprised of 50 to 60 percent water that needs to be replenished daily. Drink at least eight full glasses of water each day, more if you are exercising. Also, drink more water initially if you are still consuming beverages with caffeine, sugar or alcohol, as these chemicals cause dehydration. For variety and to spice up your water, add a lemon, lime or orange slice for flavor. Or drink the bottled water instilled with the essence of fruit.

Sparkling waters

You may drink them in place of still water if they contain less than 50 milligrams of sodium.

Caffeine-free herbal teas

You can count these as part of your water intake as long as they are not diuretic teas.

Decaffeinated coffee

If you like to drink coffee, drink water-processed decaffeinated coffee with organic whole cream. Both milk and half-and-half contain milk sugar (lactose). You may have a small amount of raw organic milk in your coffee. Do not use half-and-half because it is filled with other chemicals. This is not considered part of your essential water intake.

Vegetable juices

You can have wheat grass, spinach and/or celery juice, or any other juice you can come up with that is made from nonstarchy vegetables.

Carrot and tomato juices

Only drink on the Maintenance Plan because they contain too much sugar for the Healing Plan.

Real fruit juices

You can have real fruit juices one to three times a week as long as you are on the Maintenance Plan and exercise consistently. However, it is better to eat the fruit rather than drink it because the fiber in the fruit lowers the amount of sugar entering your body. However, if you feel like drinking something other than water, real fruit juices can be an alternative, but you must dilute them—four parts juice to one part water. Do not drink more than two glasses of diluted juice daily.

Fruit smoothies

You can have fruit smoothies one to three times a week on the maintenance plan but you must add in protein powder (not soy) or another protein source. Remember to count these as carbohydrates. Do not drink smoothies in place of a meal; do not add in frozen yogurt, sherbet, sorbet or ice cream; and do not drink more than eight ounces in one day.

What to Avoid

Milk

It is best to avoid drinking milk because it contains a great deal of hidden sugar in the form of lactose. If you are on the Maintenance Plan and want to drink milk, use raw organic whole milk because the fats in it will help slow the absorption of the sugar in the milk so that the body can process it better. If you cannot tolerate the taste of whole milk, try diluting it with water. Do not drink more than one glass of milk a day.

Caffeinated beverages

Avoid all beverages with caffeine unless you are using them as self-medication in the Healing Plan. Change all sodas, diet sodas and other caffeinated beverages to coffee or teas. Caffeinated green tea is better than black tea, which is better than coffee. The equivalent of one cup of tea or coffee a day will not break your program.

Alcohol

Avoid alcohol, but if you must drink it, drink red wine or dark beer and keep it to half of a glass or one beer per day. Do not save up the equivalent of your daily drink to have it all at once during one night. In other words, you should not drink three and a half glasses of wine or seven beers once a week.

What Not to Drink

High-fructose beverages

Avoid all beverages with high-fructose corn syrup. Fructose, a sugar found in fruits and vegetables, is more damaging to cells than white sugar when it is ingested in high amounts. Fructose is found naturally in low amounts in fruits and some vegetables, but in very high amounts in high-fructose corn syrup. Read the labels and stay away from fructose and high-fructose corn syrup sweetened products.

Artificially sweetened beverages

Avoid all beverages with artificial sweeteners. Aspartame, saccharine, sucralose, acesulfam-K and other artificial sugars all damage the cells of your body. Keep these toxic chemicals out of your system because they will age you faster.

Prepackaged vegetable juices

Do not drink prepackaged vegetable juices in cans because they usually contain too much salt.

FOODS TO AVOID

You now know which beverages to avoid or not drink. The next few pages are the foods to stop eating altogether.

Do Not Eat These Sugars and Desserts

Banana chips
Brown sugar
Candy
Caramel or other
   flavored popcorn
Cocoa
Coffeecake
Dessert toppings
Doughnuts
Eclairs
Frosting
Frozen desserts

Fruit leathers
Granola and other
   snack bars
Ice cream
Milk shakes
Pastries
Processed yogurt
   (nonfat or flavored
   yogurt with artificial
   sweetners or
   sugar added)

Protein bars (with
   man-made chemicals)
Pudding
Sherbet
Strudel
Sweet rolls
Syrups (fudge,
   corn, high-fructose
   corn, malt, maple,
   sorghum, butter-
   scotch or caramel)
Toaster pastries
White sugar

Do Not Eat These Processed Snack Foods and Breads

Beef jerky
Corn nuts
Meat-based sticks
Pork skins

Sesame sticks
Trail mix packaged
   with chocolate chips
   and other sweets

White hamburger
   and hot dog buns

Do Not Eat Condiments That Contain Sugar and Chemical Additives

Barbecue sauces
Fish sauces
Gravies
Hoisin sauce

Ketchup
Meat extender
Meat tenderizer
Oyster sauce

Relishes
Sweet pickles
Worcestershire

Do Not Eat Foods That Contain Damaged Fats, Chemicals and/or Sugar

Bottled salad dressings
Buttermilk
Cream substitutes
Cream containing chemicals
Deep-fat-fried foods
Half-and-half
High-fat meats that have been
  cooked at high temperatures
Hydrogenated oils
Imitation mayonnaise
Imitation sour cream

Lard/shortening
Margarine
Nondairy creamers
Palm oil
Pressurized whipped cream
  and dessert toppings
Processed foods and fast
  foods using hydrogenated oils
Rancid fats
Sandwich spreads

Do Not Eat Highly Processed Meat and Sausages

Barbecue loaf
Beer salami
Beerwurst
Beerwurst salami
Bologna
Corned beef loaf

Honey loaf
Honey-roll sausage
Lebanon bologna
Luxury loaf
Mother's loaf
Pastrami

Peppered loaf
Pepperoni
Picnic loaf
Pork headcheese
Salami
Vienna sausage

STAPLE FOODS

Here are some sample staple food choices that will lead to a healthy diet. Keeping your cupboards stocked with basic, healthy food staples will help you follow the Schwarzbein Principle Program to the best of your ability. If you are having problems finding acceptable food sources, please visit my Web site for the latest Healthy Products List at *www.schwarzbeinprinciple.com.*

Protein

Chicken

Cornish game hens

Cottage cheese
(organic low-fat or regular)

Eggs

Fish (only keep for a day or two)

Goat cheese

Lean cuts of beef, lamb and pork

Nitrate-free chicken or turkey
sausages

String cheese (part skim mozzarella)

Turkey

Real Carbohydrates

Complex:

Canned or fresh beans

Grains (barley, brown rice, buckwheat, bulgar, couscous, oatmeal,
popcorn kernels, quinoa)

Hummus (no additives or preservatives)

Plain, organic whole-milk yogurt or reduced-fat yogurt (no sugar
added)

Starchy vegetables (artichoke, corn, jicama, lima beans, peas, potato,
yam, squash, sweet potato)

Simple:

Fresh or frozen fruit

Man-made Carbohydrates

Whole grain or corn tortillas

Whole grain or rice bread

Whole grain or rice crackers

Fats and Oils
Butter
Coconut oil
Mayonnaise (organic, without added sugar, with pure-pressed or
  expeller-pressed oils)
Olive oil
Salad dressing (organic, without added sugar, with pure-pressed or
  expeller-pressed oils)

Healthy Fats That Contain Carbohydrates
Avocado
Nut butters
Raw nuts and seeds

Vegetables
Herbal teas
Fresh herbs and spices
Organic nonstarchy vegetables

Supplements

In addition to nutritional and diet changes, here are four core supplements that I recommend for everyone who is beginning my program.

- **A good twice-a-day multivitamin and mineral.**
- **Extra omega-3 fatty acids** to help with a variety of chemical reactions in the body.
- **Stress B complex** if you have a lot of stress, are extremely busy, drink alcohol or caffeine, or have mood disorders.
- **Calcium and magnesium** at bedtime if you do not sleep well or don't eat enough vegetables.

These are the supplements that I recommend for those with a healthy metabolism who are not under large amounts of stress. If you have a damaged metabolism, some of the following supplements are recommended to help the body function better by reversing oxidation, improving mood and energy, decreasing cravings for toxic chemicals and/or helping your body build lean body tissue and burn fat better.

———————— Additional General Supplements ————————

- **Carnitine**, an amino acid that helps burn fats for energy, improves mood and lowers triglyceride levels.
- **Carnosine**, an amino acid derivative that helps block damage from oxidation.
- **Chromium** (not a picolinate form) to help with insulin problems such as diabetes, heart disease, high blood pressure and obesity.
- **Coenzyme Q-10**, an antioxidant to protect against heart disease and raise energy and mood. This is a must if you are taking statin drugs for cholesterol.

- **Glutamine,** an amino acid that helps with carbohydrate cravings and heals the intestinal lining.
- **Lipoic acid,** a strong antioxidant that helps the body repair and improve energy use. Important in treating insulin resistant conditions.
- **N-acetyl cysteine,** an amino acid derivation that is a very strong antioxidant. Very important in detoxification involving your liver and lungs.
- **Taurine,** an amino acid to improve insulin sensitivity and help rid the body of excess water.
- **Vitamin C,** an antioxidant to improve immunity and help under times of stress. A must if you smoke.
- **Vitamin E (as mixed tocopherols),** a strong antioxidant for heart and brain health, especially if you choose to smoke.

———————— Additional Calming Supplements ————————

- **5-HTP,** an amino acid that becomes serotonin.
- **GABA,** a calming neurotransmitter good for turning off brain noise.
- **Inositol,** a B vitamin that helps increase serotonin function.
- **Lavender essential oils,** an herb that calms your brain.
- **L-theanine,** amino acid found in green tea that is very calming.
- **Krill oil,** omega-3 already in its phospholipid form to help with PMS.
- **Phosphatydal serine,** an orthomolecular molecule that lowers cortisol levels.
- **Zinc,** a mineral that decreases sympathetic flow. The sympathetic nervous system is the part of the autonomic nervous system that keeps you hyper-vigilant and alert.

—————— Additional Fat Burning Supplements ——————

- **Branched-chain amino acids,** leucine, isoleucine and valine.
- **Epigallocatechin gallate (EGCg),** a green tea extract.

—————— Additional Digestive Aids ——————

- **Betaine HCL** is hydrochloric acid. It works by activating your own digestive enzymes.
- **Digestive enzymes** help you digest your foods and help with absorption.

I have not recommended any *specific* doses because I don't necessarily want you to take exactly what I write, *nor everything that I recommend.* You need to work with your healthcare provider in determining which of these supplements are best for you. Please visit my Web site (*www.schwarzbeinprinciple.com*) for more information regarding supplements.

Stress Management

If you cannot get rid of all your stresses (and most of us can't), you need to learn how to manage them better. By managing your stresses, you slow the using side of your metabolism. By getting enough uninterrupted sleep, you provide your body with the time it needs to rebuild.

The most common mistakes regarding stress and sleep issues are the following:

- Not acknowledging how harmful stress is to your health;
- Not recognizing that being busy is a stress;
- Not realizing that stress makes you gain fat weight, and instead of working on eliminating the stress, you eat less;
- Not taking the time to sleep;

• Accepting that it is okay to wake up during the night so you don't address this problem;
• Not discussing your sleep problems with your health-care provider; and
• Taking sleeping pills instead of sleep resetting medication.

The Schwarzbein Principle Program recognizes the importance of finding a way to manage your stresses better. If you are under tremendous amounts of emotional stress due to financial, personal or work pressures, it is usually impossible for you to make or maintain the necessary nutrition and lifestyle changes I am advocating. Therefore, you need to manage your stress or you can never be fully healthy. This will not only help slow the using-up side of your metabolism, it will allow you to eliminate other bad habits. After all, stress—or more accurately the desire to calm yourself down and feel less anxious and depressed— is one of the main causes of eating poorly, overexercising, and using alcohol, tobacco and drugs. Also, stress keeps you from getting a good night's sleep.

This program does not offer a separate way for you to fix emotional problems, but it recognizes the importance of doing so. If eating and sleeping well and taking HRT doesn't help, and if you are too distraught, you will have to do some emotional work *as part of the program* before you completely master this step and reap all the health benefits. You should talk through your emotional issues with family, clergy or friends. If this doesn't work, seek professional help.

The Power of Sleep

Not sleeping enough is a physical stress that impacts your health. And, if you do not sleep well, you will not be able to handle your emotional stresses well. By working on getting enough sleep as the

first step of your stress management process, you take away a physical stress and give your body the rest it needs to confront and conquer your emotional stresses.

If you have not been sleeping well for years, you may find yourself getting more tired as you catch up on your missed sleep. This is normal and, if it happens, unavoidable. You need to realize that this is part of the catching-up-with-sleep process and give yourself permission to be tired and sleep more as needed. The fatigue will go away once you have caught up with sleep.

Getting a Great Night's Sleep

The definition of a good night's rest is being able to fall asleep easily and stay asleep for at least eight hours (preferably more). If you wake up or get up once to urinate and are able to go right back to sleep, that is okay. But great sleep is when you do not wake up at all. You need to work on getting a *great* night's sleep! For most, this is the easiest part of stress management to work on. Here are the steps:

- Give yourself enough time to sleep and change your sleep environment.
- Use lavender essential oil to relax.
- Add supplements as needed.
- Try a sleep resetting medication.
- As a last resort, add a selective serotonin reuptake inhibitor (SSRI) drug.

Make the Time to Sleep and Change Your Poor Sleep Environment

Start by making the time to sleep. You do this by getting to bed earlier so that you have enough time to sleep at least a full eight hours. Make sure that your environment is favorable to sleep—no noises, very dark, comfortable mattress, and the room is the right

temperature for you. Try to wind down an hour or so before bedtime so that you are not too wired to fall asleep, and last but not least, keep animals, children and snoring significant others away (as much as possible) until you can establish a constant sleep pattern.

Here is a list of reasons you may not be sleeping well and some commonsense solutions:

Are you falling asleep easily but find yourself waking up in the middle of the night or too early in the morning?

- Stop drinking or decrease your **alcohol** intake as described in step 3.
- Make sure you are **eating well**. Do not skip meals or snacks and make sure you are eating the right portion sizes and the correct balance of protein and carbohydrates at each mealtime.
- **Menopause** is a common cause of sleeping problems. In fact most women wake up between 2 and 4 A.M. when their estradiol levels are out of balance. Check with your physician to see if you need to start taking HRT or have your estradiol or progesterone prescription adjusted. If you are taking HRT but are not on an estradiol and/or progesterone preparation, ask your physician to change your prescription. There are many different delivery systems available, from pills and patches to sublingual troches (lozenges) and sublingual drops. Not every delivery system works the same for every woman. Trial and error will help you find the system that works best for you.
- Excessive **emotional stress** can keep you from getting a good night's sleep. Acknowledge there is a problem and seek help if needed.

Are you waking up in the night with a full bladder?

- Watch your **bedtime fluid intake.**
- Evaluate your **diabetes program.** You may be waking up at night to urinate because your blood sugar levels are too high or too low.
- Men, you may have an enlarged **prostate.** Have this checked by your primary care provider.

Are you too "buzzed" to settle down in bed?

- *Don't drink **caffeinated beverages** in the afternoon or evening. You may not think it is affecting you, but it probably is.
- *Don't run around finishing chores** and staying busy right before bedtime. Do something relaxing before bed like taking a warm bath, meditating or reading.
- *Overexercising,** especially late in the day, can overstimulate your body and keep you from feeling tired even when you are.
- *Refined sugar** is a stimulant. If you must eat it, try eating it earlier in the day. When you are able, get off of refined sugar as much as possible.

Do you have trouble falling asleep?

- **Don't power nap.** It is better to sleep at night and be awake during the day. However, a short nap between 3 and 4 P.M. will not break this program unless it keeps you from getting to sleep at a decent hour or staying asleep at night.
- Work on **stress management** techniques. One technique you can try is to keep a pen and paper by your bedside and write down all the thoughts running through your head that may be keeping you from relaxing. Sometimes by writing your list down, you can get it to stay out of your brain for the night. The same applies to waking

up in the middle of the night with 101 worries and "to do" thoughts. Write them down so that you may fall back to sleep.

- *You may have a **zinc deficiency** keeping you from sleeping well. Take the zinc challenge (see pg. 96) and start replacement if needed.

Are you groggy in the morning and don't feel rested?

- Give yourself **enough hours in bed.** Try not to wake up to alarm clocks, but get to bed early enough that you will wake up naturally eight or more hours later.
- Try to cut back on your use of **tobacco products** and taper off them completely if possible.

Are you experiencing physical problems or changes?

- If you have **acid reflux,** sleep with your head elevated and discuss this problem with your primary care physician. One of the safest and most inexpensive prescription medications on the market is sulcrafate (brand name Carafate). It works by coating the lining of your intestines and protecting them against acid damage. Even taking one 1000 mg pill at night can be lifesaving. I recommend this above any other acid reflux medication on the market today. Of couse, evaluating and fixing the cause of acid reflux is essential.
- If **allergies** are waking you up at night, try quercetin, bromelain, magnesium and methylsulfonylmethane (MSM). If these don't work, consult your physician regarding medication for allergies. Try to avoid those with cortisone or adrenalinelike action.
- **Grinding your teeth** can keep you from getting a good night's sleep. Have your teeth evaluated for signs of wear and tear.
- If you are in **pain,** get help. Don't just self-medicate. See a chiropractor, physical therapist or acupuncturist to see if your pain can be managed without narcotics and analgesics.

- **Sleep apnea** is a medical condition where you stop breathing for an extended time interval when you are sleeping. A common symptom is excessive snoring. Have a significant other check to see that you do not stop breathing through the night. Or better yet, have a sleep study.

Are you taking medication?

- Consult with your physician and read the package drug insert on **antidepressant medication** to make sure the antidepressant you are using is not the reason you are sleeping so poorly.
- The long-term use of diazepam, lorazepam and alprazolam (**anti-anxiety drugs**) and other drugs of this class disrupt REM sleep. The same is true for **sleeping pills.** Discuss how to get off these medications with your primary care physician or try switching to a sleep-resetting drug, such as Desyrel.
- All types of **chemical birth control** can disrupt your sleep. This is true even if you have been using them for a long time before your sleep problems began. Consider changing to barrier methods such as condoms, cervical caps and the diaphragm.
- Make sure you are taking the right type and dose of thyroid hormone replacement for **hypothyroidism** (an underactive thyroid condition) or the right medications for **hyperthyroidism** (an overactive thyroid problem). Discuss this with your primary care physician.
- Ask your pharmacist whether any **over-the-counter medicines** you are taking, including herbal products, contain any chemical that may disturb sleep.
- Ask your pharmacist or physician whether any **prescription medicines** you are taking contain any chemical that may disturb sleep.

---

*Do you have a new baby?

• There is not much that can be done about this one except to share the nighttime duties with your partner. Napping is a good way to catch up on some of the missed sleep. However, as soon as you can, you should resume your normal sleep habits.

* These issues may also cause you to wake up in the middle of the night. In the case of the new baby, it's almost a guarantee.

Lavender Oil

A few drops of a high-grade essential lavender oil can be placed on a piece of cloth or handkerchief (some brands can be placed directly on your upper lip; check the label). Breathe in deeply through your nose and see if this helps you relax enough to fall asleep. You can try this again if you wake up in the night. Be sure to use a certified organic, 100 percent pure lavender oil.

Other relaxing herbs are chamomile or passion flower. Stay away from products that contain valerian root and kava kava. These are as potent as some drugs.

Adding Supplements

If changing your sleep habits doesn't work and lavender oil is not enough, it's time to add supplements. Start with taking the following supplements in this order. Not everyone will need to take all of them at the same time. Use calcium with magnesium first and add sequential supplements as needed. Start with low doses of each and work your way up to the higher doses as needed. Make sure to discuss these recommendations with your primary care physician.

1. Calcium (500 mg to 1000 mg) and magnesium (250 mg to 500 mg) at bedtime. If you get constipated lower the calcium dose; if you get loose bowel movements it is from too much magnesium. In general, calcium is needed in a dose that is twice that of the magnesium dose.

2. Add 5 -HTP (50 mg to 200 mg) or L-tryptophan (500 mg to 2000 mg) at bedtime next. Higher doses should be supervised by your health-care practitioner.
   Note: Do not use 5-HTP or L-tryptophan if you are taking anti-depressants unless supervised by a physician.

3. Add inositol (500 mg to 3000 mg).

4. Adding phosphatidyl serine (100 mg to 200 mg) at bedtime is really helpful for those whose sympathetic nervous system is overactive. Common causes of overactive sympathetic nervous system are past or present stress and having burned out adrenal glands.

5. Add taurine (500 mg to 1000 mg) at night to help calm you down.

6. If you are low in zinc, you need to take zinc in the morning and evening. Zinc (25 mg to 30 mg) at bedtime helps calm you down. Only take extra zinc if you are zinc depleted (see box, pg. 96).

7. Adding gamma amino butyric acid (GABA) (500 mg to 1000 mg) at night or earlier helps turn off the constant chatter in your head. Or you can use this if you wake up at night and cannot get back to sleep because you cannot turn your thoughts off, but try lavender oil first. It is less expensive and has less possible negative effects.

NOTE: *If you begin having vivid, colorful dreams or night-mares it is most likely the inositol, 5-HTP, L-tryptophan or GABA.*

The Zinc Challenge

Zinc is an important element in the body. Among other things, it helps maintain a healthy immune system, build new tissues, repair leaky gut, improve digestion, increase insulin sensitivity and create healthy skin. The zinc challenge will help determine if you are low in zinc. Do not take this test on an empty stomach. Remember that it is important to take zinc with vitamin B_2 because they work together. A deficiency of vitamin B_2 can lead to a zinc-deficient result on this test. You can buy the zinc challenge liquid and zinc pills off my Web site at *www.schwarzbeinprinciple.com.*

1. Take two capfuls of the zinc challenge liquid and hold it in your mouth for at least 30 seconds. If it has a strong metallic taste spit it out. If it doesn't taste bad you can swallow it. It is only zinc.
2. If you have a strong metallic taste, you have adequate zinc. You do not need to add more zinc to your vitamin regimen.
3. If you have a slight rusty nail or fuzzy mouth taste, you are slightly low in zinc. Take zinc replacement of 25 mg per capsule, one capsule morning and night. Rechallenge yourself every one to two weeks and decrease to one pill in the evening when you have a strong metallic taste.
4. If the zinc challenge liquid tastes like water, you are zinc deficient. Take the zinc challenge liquid (one tablespoon) twice a day. When you have a strong metallic taste of zinc, switch to the zinc pills and take one pill morning and night. Rechallenge yourself every one to two weeks and if you continue to taste the zinc as a strong metallic taste, decrease to one pill in the evening. Or you can take the zinc pills, one or two pills twice a day, and rechallenge yourself with the liquid zinc every one to two weeks, making the change to one pill in the evening when appropriate.

Sleep Resetting Medication

Though I am mostly in favor of not taking prescription medications, some of you will not be able to get a great night's sleep without help. If you are in this predicament, it is better to take medication than it is to forgo sleep. However, I want you to take a sleep resetting medication not a sleeping pill.

There are sleep resetting medications and there are sleeping pills. Do not confuse them; they are not the same things. Sleep resetting medications, unlike sleeping pills, are not addictive and help to re-establish normal sleep-wake cycles.

If needed, try taking Desyrel 25 mg to 100 mg at bedtime. Desyrel is a drug and does have side effects. The most common are dry mouth, grogginess and headaches. Therefore, you should always start at the lowest dose and work your way up slowly. Take 25 mg (if you are very sensitive to medications, you can start off taking 12.5 mg), and if after two to three days there is no effect, increase to 50 mg. If you need more than 100 mg at night to sleep, you are using this medication as an antidepressant. It would be better to stay with lower doses of Desyrel (25 mg to 100 mg) at night and add an SSRI in the morning* as needed.

Remember, this is not a typical sleeping pill so do not expect it to work the first night you take it. However, it will knock some people out for the night, and you may or may not feel groggy the next morning. Feeling tired in the morning is not a good reason to stop taking this medication. If you are sleeping through the night and waking up tired, try tapering down by 12.5 mg at a time until you are sleeping through the night and are not so tired.

Some of you will be tired because you are catching up with sleep. This is a normal response to reversing sleep deprivation. It is okay to feel tired. If you have too much to do in the morning, drink caffeinated tea or coffee to keep you going. It is extremely important to re-establish the normal wake-sleep patterns: awake in the day, and asleep at night.

---

*I recommend that you try taking SAM-e or L-tryptophan during the day along with the recommended supplements for a damaged metabolism to boost your serotonin levels before adding in an SSRI.

SSRI

As a final resort, and I mean *final* resort, you may need a selective serotonin reuptake inhibitor (SSRI) medication to help you sleep. There are many of these on the market, *but discuss their use with your primary care physician before taking any medication.* Do not be ashamed to take SSRI in the short term to reset your sleep cycle. If you cannot sleep with the first four recommendations, you have dug yourself into a deep metabolic hole and will need further drug assistance to help you out of it. As long as you are improving your nutrition and lifestyle habits while on these types of medication, you decrease the risk of doing irreversible damage. Ideally, you will be able to come off them within the year.

Managing Stress

Stress is defined as the psychological strain that you encounter on a day-to-day basis. Ideally, it would be great to eliminate all the things that stress you out. However, this is not realistic. Instead of focusing on eliminating your stress, you need to learn how to manage it better. A good night's sleep is the first step. The second step is to make sure you have enough daily downtime. Downtime is when your brain is *not* being bombarded with 1,001 different thoughts or tasks. Downtime is important because it is one of the times that your brain rests and rebuilds. The other time is during restful sleep.

The idea behind downtime is to quiet your brain and fill yourself with joy. As strange as this may seem, this can be accomplished while doing simple household tasks such as folding laundry or washing dishes. Others prefer more recognized stress reducers such as taking baths, getting massages or having body treatments like facials and pedicures. Playing a musical instrument or singing works for some, while reading books and watching sitcoms works for others. Get to know

yourself and what it takes to turn off your brain. Nothing is a waste of time if it lets your brain rest.

If you cannot find time for yourself on a day-to-day basis or cannot relax when you do find the time, I recommend that you find a stress management technique that suits your personality and implement it as part of your health routine. Deep breathing, visualization, meditation and restorative yoga are examples of such techniques. Use these techniques in addition to your other downtime methods.

There are also stress management experts who can help you get back in touch with your body. This is called "somatization work." These various techniques help lower your sympathetic (stimulating) outflow and increase your parasympathetic (calming) outflow.

Here are some hints that may help you manage stress better:

- Love can be a very powerful stress reducer. Surround yourself with people who calm you down just by their very presence.
- Learn to manage your time effectively.
- Decide what is important. Learn to schedule your priorities.
- Enjoy the moment.
- Love yourself.
- Learn to breathe deeply and correctly.
- Find a relaxing exercise you enjoy.
- Develop a positive mental attitude.
- Do not take life too seriously. Laughter is very healing.
- Pick your battles carefully. If a point is not important in the long run, let it go.
- Get a massage.
- Engage in an activity that allows your brain to rest.
- Allow yourself enough time to sleep each night.
- Do not make several life changes at one time (if you can avoid it). Ending a relationship, moving to a new house or city, changing jobs, or losing loved ones are very stressful situations. If you cannot avoid such a situation, realize how extremely stressed you are

and make other changes in your life to help you counter the stress.

- Take a vacation.
- Take time with friends.
- Take up yoga.
- Slow down by not interrupting others. Practice waiting in line, driving in the slow lane and eating slowly.
- Give love to your pets.
- Learn to meditate.
- If you believe in God, pray.
- Set realistic goals for yourself and others.
- Take a long, hot bubble bath!
- Surround yourself with beauty, such as flowers, scented candles, artwork and anything else that appeals to your senses.
- Organize your environment to unclutter your mind.
- Make a "To Do" list and cross off each item as you complete it.
- Attend a stress management seminar, read a good book or listen to tapes on the subject of stress.
- Ask for help. It is not shameful to seek advice from professionals. After all, your health is at stake!

Minis

Minis are breathing techniques to help you relax anywhere and anytime. They don't require any audiovisual equipment, don't cost anything and can be done easily by anybody. You just need yourself and a few minutes of time to do them.

Everyone can find the time in their busy lives to take a few minutes to breathe deeply. There is no valid excuse not to incorporate minis into your day. I know you will be pleased how these simple techniques can help you deal with your daily stresses better.

Here are two mini favorites:

The basics:

- Make yourself comfortable where you are or move to a quiet spot if available
- Close your eyes if the situation permits

Mini Exercise One:

- Inhale slowly and deeply
- When you exhale say the number 5 in a hushed voice or think it inside your head
- Again inhale slowly and deeply
- When you exhale say the number 4 in a hushed voice or think it inside your head
- Continue breathing in and out counting backwards to 1.
- Repeat as needed anytime and anywhere. You should notice you feel more relaxed after just 5 breaths!

Mini Exercise Two:

- Inhale slowly and deeply, then exhale slowly and let all the air back out.
- Each time you inhale think the following words "I'm grateful"
- Each time you exhale think or say the following "That life is good" or "For the Schwarzbein Principle"
- Breathe in and out, repeating these thoughts or words for at least 5 breaths. Or better yet come up with your own words on why you are grateful.

Recommended Reading and Listening for Managing Stress

There are many good books and tapes available to help you manage your stress. I have listed a few of them to help you get started.

Books

A Manual for Living, Epictetus. Harper Publishers
Being Peace, Thich Nhat Hanh. Parallax Press
Find a Quiet Corner, Nancy O'Hara. Warner Books
One Day My Soul Just Opened Up, Iyanla Vanzant. Simon & Schuster
Peace Is Every Step, Thich Nhat Hanh. Bantam Books
Stress Management Made Simple, Jay Winner, M.D. Blue Fountain Press
Succulent Wild Woman: Dancing With Your Wonder-Full Self, Sark. Simon & Schuster
The Artist's Way, Julia Cameron. G. P. Putnam's Sons
The Creative Journal: The Art of Finding Yourself, Lucia Capacchione, Ph.D. Newcastle Publishing
The Little Book of Joy: An Interpretive Journal for Thoughts, Prayers, and Wishes, Bill Zimmerman. Hazelden Information Education
The Power of Optimism, Alan Loy McGinnis. HarperCollins
The Quieting Reflex, Charles Stroebel, M.D., Ph.D. Berkeley Publishing Group
The Relaxation Response, Herbert Benson, M.D. Avon Books
The Simple Abundance Companion, Sarah Ban Breathnach. Warner Books
The Woman's Book of Courage: Meditations for Empowerment & Peace of Mind, Sue Patton Thoele. Conari Press
You Must Relax, Edmund Jacobson. McGraw-Hill
The Taming of the Chew: A Holistic Guide to Stopping Compulsive Eating, Denise Lamothe, Psy.D., H.H.D. Penguin Books (This book is important for anyone who is stressed from his or her eating disorder.)

Tapes

Affirmations, Belleruth Naparstek
Experiencing Stress, Belleruth Naparstek
General Wellness, Belleruth Naparstek

Check out my Web site at *www.schwarzbeinprinciple.com.* I will update the book and tape lists as I discover new options.

theschwarzbeinprinciple
THE
PROGRAM

losing weight the healthy way
an easy, 5-step, no-nonsense approach

Diana Schwarzbein, M.D.

Health Communications, Inc.
Deerfield Beach, Florida

www.bcibooks.com

Seven

Toxic Chemicals

> **The Schwarzbein Way:**
> *Eliminate or drastically reduce the use of tobacco, alcohol, refined sugar, artificial sugar, caffeine and medicines, but don't stop cold turkey. Wean yourself from the specific chemicals you crave through addressing the reasons you are using them to self medicate.*

Toxic chemicals, such as refined sugars, alcohol, nicotine, artificial sugars, caffeine and many medical drugs, accelerate the turnover of chemicals and cells in your body and therefore speed up the normal aging process. By using less or avoiding them completely, you will let your body rebuild more efficiently. However, some of these toxic chemicals will need to be continued until your metabolism is healed significantly.

The most common mistakes regarding chemicals are the following:

• Using caffeine, nicotine, sugar or alcohol to make yourself feel

better or "more alert" without improving eating, stress and sleep habits;

- Trying to stop using these chemicals before changing the reasons you are taking them in the first place (increased stress, lack of sleep, poor nutrition, etc.); and
- Substituting artificial sugar for refined sugar with the flawed notion that ingesting less calories is better than the bad effects of these toxic chemicals;
- Taking medications without working on nutrition and lifestyle habits;
- Avoiding the use of medication if nothing else is working.

In general, you use toxic chemicals to feel better or get more things done when you are either too stressed, overexercising or not eating properly. Toxic chemicals cause your body to break down, so when you ingest any toxic chemical, you trigger the pathways in your body that access energy and other substances that help with mood, concentration and a feeling of well-being. That is why all toxic chemicals are addicting; they artificially make you feel better.

You can't just stop using these chemicals cold turkey without changing the reasons that you need them in the first place or you will fall apart either mentally, physically or both. Furthermore, stopping these chemicals abruptly may make it impossible for you to adopt the necessary lifestyle changes that will help you balance your metabolism. Don't do this to yourself. You will only feel like a failure. The road to health is a process. If you work on the underlying problems first, the need for these chemicals will go away. Only then can you taper off them successfully.

One of the most important habits to change in order to be able to get off of toxic chemicals is how you eat. You need to eat balanced meals throughout the day. If you find yourself uncontrollably craving a toxic chemical such as sugar, nicotine or alcohol, you need to give

into your craving—but you must continue to eat well. If you don't eat enough to rebuild, you will continue *to need* your toxic chemical.

Sleep is another important habit that can help you get off toxic chemicals. One of the reasons you are ingesting many of these chemicals is to have more energy. However, the best way to have more energy is to rebuild energy during sleep, not break down healthy tissues by ingesting toxic chemicals.

Always keep in mind that getting off toxic chemicals *is not* the first step in healing your metabolism. Eating, sleeping well and managing your stress comes first, and if you need to self-medicate for this to happen, you should stay on some of your toxic chemicals a while longer.

If you have diabetes, heart disease or high blood pressure disease, or you have had blood clots, a heart attack or stroke, getting off of tobacco, alcohol and refined sugar is a priority. As an intermediate solution replace them as quickly as you can with less harmful chemicals. Substitute nicotine for tobacco and caffeinated coffee, black tea or green tea and/or Stevia for alcohol and refined sugars. If you are very addicted to alcohol, try GABA and glutamine and switch heavy liquor to dark beer or red wine. If you are very addicted to refined sugar, try eating more berries and grapefruit with organic whole fat whipping cream and small amounts of bitter, dark chocolate instead. As soon as you can, begin to taper off nicotine, alcohol and sugars completely.

Here is a list of toxic chemicals in order of most to least harmful. As much as possible, try to exchange a worse (higher on the list) toxic chemical for one further down on the list. Never go the other way around. In the best-case scenario, you end up drinking a lot of green tea instead of smoking cigarettes or drinking alcohol.

Though it is best to get off of all chemicals that cause your body to use itself up, if you have a healthy metabolism, small amounts of red wine, dark beer, fruit juice, milk and organic whole-food desserts made with real sugar will not break your program.

Although most prescription drugs, including over-the-counter drugs, are more harmful than caffeinated beverages, they are listed last because you need to work with your physician and cannot exchange them for other toxic chemicals.

Toxic Chemicals, in order from worst to (relative) best

- Illicit drugs and narcotics
- Tobacco/nicotine
- Alcohol
- Artificial sugars including sucralose, aspartame, acesulfam-K and saccharine, alone or in food and beverages, including diet sodas, even if they are decaffeinated
- Refined sugars, such as sucrose, fructose, maltose, dextrose, maltodextrin, polydextrose, corn syrup and high fructose corn syrup found in (among many other food products) sodas and sugary foods
- Additives, chemical preservatives and other fake chemicals
- Caffeinated beverages like coffee, yerba mate and teas
- Over-the-counter medications
- Prescription medications

Illicit Drugs and Narcotics

These types of drugs are harmful in many ways. They alter your body chemistry and affect your decision making. They decrease your appetite

and therefore keep you from eating well. They "work" by getting your body to release its own natural feel-good chemicals in much higher quantities than needed until you run out of them, leaving you listless, depressed and in perpetual pain. These are very addicting substances and should be avoided.

Tobacco/Nicotine

Tobacco is harmful because it causes oxidative damage to cells, cholesterol and brain tissue. Nicotine is a stimulant that causes your body to use itself up more than build. It also decreases appetite and increases blood pressure and heart rate. Together, tobacco and nicotine cause cancers, heart attacks, strokes, emphysema, dementia, depression, allergies, acid reflux and osteoporosis, among many other problems. Nicotine alone is less harmful. If you can, switch to nicotine only products now.

Alcohol

Alcohol is a chemical that directly causes cell death. It has been linked to many cancers, including colon, breast and prostate. The sugar in alcoholic beverages increases the release of insulin, causing the sugar to be preferentially converted into fats. All forms of alcohol make diabetes, cholesterol, blood pressure, established heart disease and fat weight worse. Red wine and dark beer are the least harmful types of alcohol. If you can, switch all alcohol to red wine or dark beer now.

Artificial Sweeteners

All artificial sweeteners are harmful because they are unnatural—your body does not need them, nor can it use them to rebuild with.

They cause chemical and hormonal imbalances that increase the turnover of cells and stimulate your appetite for further toxic chemical ingestion. It is better to use small amounts of organic honey, xylitol or Stevia than it is to use any artificial sweetener. Switch over as soon as you can.

Refined Sugars

Refined white or brown sugars include sucrose, fructose, maltose, dextrose, maltodextrin, polydextrose, corn syrup and high fructose corn syrup. Eating and drinking sugar and sugary foods is detrimental because it oxidizes cells, chemicals and tissues. It depletes your body of "feel-good chemicals." And it triggers proinflammatory chemicals to be secreted and produced in higher quantities. That is why sugar increases the risk of the degenerative diseases of aging as well as symptoms such as heartburn, arthritis pain, headaches, depression and agitation. Don't be fooled by milk and fruit juice. Though they are better than other sugary drinks, they contain a lot of hidden refined sugars, too.

As you begin to eat regular meals and snacks, you will notice a decrease in your need for refined sugars. If you get a craving, give in early and choose fruits, organic honey, bitter dark chocolate and whole ingredient desserts over junk food. However, you may not count this sugar binge as a meal or snack. It is through consistent eating of balanced foods that you will be able to get off of sugar completely.

Additives, Chemical Preservatives and Other Fake Chemicals

MSG and other preservatives and additives are man-made chemicals that interfere with the normal chemical signaling between cells. Fake fats such as Olestra interfere with the absorption of fat-soluble vitamins and healthy fats. Carbohydrate and fat blockers block the

absorption of healthy fats and real carbohydrates. Again, these products are unnatural—not found in nature—so your body can't use them. None of these chemicals are addicting, so you can stop using them now.

Caffeine

Caffeinated products affect the body by decreasing its ability to metabolize and dispose of adrenaline. High levels of adrenaline give you energy, but cause the body to use up its chemicals faster than it rebuilds them. Caffeinated drinks, in order of worst (never drink) to best (*okay in small amounts because of their antioxidant benefits), are:

Diet sodas
Sodas
Caffeinated waters
*Yerba Mate
*Coffee
*Black tea
*Green tea

Start to switch to a better form of caffeine now. NOTE: The decaffeinated equivalent of each selection is better to drink as long as it is not chemically processed. Remember that you may need to use caffeine to help you heal your metabolism, so do not try stopping all caffeine before you are ready (refer to the Healing or Maintenance Plans).

Over-the-Counter Drugs

Most over-the-counter medications used for pain relief, heartburn, cough and colds, constipation, headaches, muscle aches and pains, and other symptoms are man-made chemicals that have no place in normal physiological functions. Although they are sold over the counter, they are still drugs with side effects. Even worse, these drugs aren't helping your body, they are simply masking the symptoms of more serious body problems. Some common drugs and their most serious side effects are listed below.

- **Acetaminophen** ... can cause liver damage
- **Acid blockers** . . . can decrease your ability to digest and absorb proteins, leading to malnourishment
- **Antacids contain aluminum and sometimes magnesium** ... can cause brain damage and calcium imbalances
- **Cough and cold medications that contain stimulants** ... can cause cardiovascular collapse
- **Laxatives containing cascara segrada** ... have been linked to increased risk of colon problems including colon cancer.
- **Nonsteroidal anti-inflammatory medications and salicylates** ... can cause kidney damage
- **Sleep aids** ... can cause further disruption to your sleep cycle, requiring that you keep taking them and depriving you of getting your needed REM sleep

Over-the-Counter Supplements

Instead of using over-the-counter drugs, try over-the counter supplements to help with symptoms such as colds, pain and headaches. Here are a few alternatives.

- **Acid reflux**—Try digestive enzymes first, and after reflux symptoms subside, add Betaine HCL acid. You can also try an artichoke extract or a product known as Digest RC that contains black radish juice, charcoal and cholic acid.
- **Allergies**—MSM, quercetin with bromelain and GLA (gamma linolenic acid, an omega-6 fatty acid found in primrose, black currant and borage oil).
- **Anti-inflammatory agents**—GLA, ginger, ginko biloba, green tea catechins and turmeric (curcumin).
- **Arthritis pain**—glucosamine and chondroitin sulfate with manganese, MSM, SAM-e, B vitamins, vitamin C or capsaicin cream or gel rubbed directly on the joint that hurts.
- **Chronic pain**—D, L, phenylalanine (the mixed D and L forms of phenylalanine), B_6 and B_{12} have been shown to protect our own pain chemicals, the endorphins.
- **Colds**—Zinc in pills, liquid and nasal gel forms as well as Immunocal (a powdered dcrink that boosts levels of a very powerful antioxidant called gluthathione) can help you fight off your cold faster. Eucalyptus essential oils can be used to open clogged nasal passages.
- **Constipation**—Oregano oil to kill off fungus, yeast and bacteria in your colon; digestive enzymes to help you digest your food; strong probiotics to recolonize with healthy bacteria. Also make sure to take a soluble fiber mix with guar gum, apple or citrus pectin, and psyllium husk. Drink plenty of water.
- **Migraine Headaches**—Ginger, feverfew, vitamin B_2, butterbur root and/or magnesium.

Prescription Medications

The prescription drugs listed below should be avoided or eliminated if possible. However, *do not stop taking any of these medications on your own*. Stopping these medications requires supervision. Work with your physician.

Cholesterol-Lowering Drugs—HMG-CoA Reductase Medicines

These drugs may increase blood sugar levels and triglyceride levels. They may also decrease the production of coenzyme Q-10 and hormones made from cholesterol such as testosterone, DHEA, cortisol, vitamin D and estradiol. Consequences may include calcium imbalances, weakness, fatigue and reduction of your sex drive. They also increase the risk of liver damage and/or muscle damage and have caused death as a result of these complications.

I am opposed to this type of drug because I believe you can lower your oxidized cholesterol (the kind that leads to increased heart attack risk) by improving your nutrition and lifestyle habits without increasing your risks for other diseases. However, if you need to stay on this type of medication until you can improve your habits, pravastatin sodium or simvastatin are the better ones to use as they have been shown to decrease the risk of a heart attack through their anti-inflammatory effects, not their cholesterol lowering ability. Make sure you are taking extra Coenzyme Q-10 if you are taking a statin drug.

There are many natural chemicals that can help normalize cholesterol levels such as carnitine, omega-3 fatty acids, tocotrienols, green tea extract, turmeric, allicin, niacin and soluble fiber. I highly recommend that you take some of these, work on your habits and get off your statin drugs as soon as possible.

Since a major cause of heart attacks is related to the amount of inflammation in your body, one simple prevention to reduce your risk is to floss your teeth daily and have your teeth cleaned regularly.

Beta-blockers

These medicines block the action of adrenaline, leading to fatigue, worsening asthma, weight gain or an inability to lose weight, and depression. The only legitimate indication for these is in the treatment of post–myocardial infarction to put the heart at rest and for treatment of arrhythmias that don't respond to other medications.

Ask your health care provider if there is a different medication such as a calcium channel blocker (CCB), an angiotensin-converting enzyme (ACE) inhibitor or an angiotensin receptor blocker (ARB) that might work for your particular medical condition.

Diuretics

Thiazide diuretics mess up your physiology by disrupting the metabolism of uric acid, electrolytes, fats and sugar. Side effects of these drugs include gout, potassium imbalances, triglyceride problems, increased blood sugar and worsening of insulin resistance. I don't believe anyone should take thiazide diuretics for any reason. There are less harmful medications for blood pressure and excess fluid retention on the market.

A great book on better drugs for high blood pressure is *What Your Doctor May Not Tell You About Hypertension,* published in 2003 by Warner Books. It also includes suggestions for supplements to lower blood pressure, too. If you need to be on a diuretic, switch to furosemide or spironolactone. Although they are usually stronger diuretics, they don't mess up your metabolism as much as thiazide diuretics do. Better still, if you are using thiazide diuretics for blood pressure problems, ask to be switched to an ACE inhibitor, an ARB medication or a CCB drug.

Sulfonylurea or Meglitinide Drugs

These two classes of drugs are used to treat the high blood-sugar levels in people with Type II diabetes by increasing insulin secretion. In so doing, they wear out your pancreas and increase your risk for

requiring life-long insulin injections. They also cause an increase in fat weight, insulin resistance and the risk of dying of a heart attack. It is better to switch to drugs that improve the action of insulin such as metformin, pioglitazone and rosioglitazone rather than continue taking these two classes of drugs that beat up on the pancreas to increase insulin secretion. It is also better to take insulin in the short term, if needed to put your pancreas at rest to rebuild, than to continue to damage your pancreas further so that you require insulin forever. I don't recommend these drugs at all because their risks outweigh their "so called" benefits.

Steroids

Steroids are cortisol derivatives. They are used as anti-inflammatory drugs for many disorders, including asthma, soft tissue injuries, connective tissue disorders and autoimmune problems. These drugs can be lifesaving, so depending on the situation, you may need to use them. The long-term use of these drugs may cause Type II diabetes, osteoporosis, suppressed immune system problems, destruction of connective tissues, osteoarthritis and heart disease, to name just a few disorders.

The goal is to get off of them as soon as you can. It is important to taper off steroids *when you can*, because they damage your metabolism. If you need to continue them, taper down to the lowest dose that works. If you have been using steroids for a long time, you need to taper off of them very slowly. It is very dangerous to come off of steroids quickly, especially if you still need them for a life-threatening illness. Always check with your physician first. The first goal is to taper down the steroid dose to one that supplies you with your daily cortisol needs. For prednisone the daily dose is around 7.5 mg, for hydrocortisone it is around 30 mg a day.

Birth Control Medication

Here is another class of drugs that I believe no woman should take. There is nothing good about these pills, pellets or vaginal tablets. Birth

control medications disrupt the sex hormone system. Since all hormones are connected, they therefore disrupt all the rest of the body's hormones, too. Alternative birth control methods are safer and can be just as effective if used correctly. Discuss the different barrier-method options with your health care practitioner and the best time to stop using this method of birth control for you. Be aware that long-term use of BCPs can lead to problems such as obesity, infertility, fibroid tumors, chronic fatigue, headaches, insomnia, high blood pressure, pulmonary embolisms, strokes, heart attacks and Type II diabetes.

If you have been using this method of birth control for a long time, when you stop you may experience numerous symptoms until your own body starts kicking in and producing your sex hormones again. You may need short-term hormone replacement therapy with bioidentical estradiol and progesterone until this system starts working properly again.

Estrogen combined with a progestin

Continuous combined therapy or suppression therapy is when you take any form of estrogen daily combined with a much higher dose of any form of progesterone, aka progestin, daily. This combination form of HRT damages your metabolism and increases your risk for the degenerative diseases of aging, as recently verified by the Women's Health Initiative (WHI). I don't advocate any woman taking HRT this way. However, please do not stop taking your therapy cold turkey or abruptly change how you are taking your hormones if you have been using this method of HRT for a long time. Progestins are stimulants so taking them continuously can be as "addicting" as any drug. If you stop too quickly, you can crash emotionally and/or physically. Though I do want you off this way of taking HRT, it is not an emergency and you don't need to suffer. If you have been taking continuous combined HRT for a long time, work with someone who knows how to transition you to bioidentical hormones taken in a cyclical manner.

Antidepressants/antianxiety

Please do *not* stop taking an antidepressant or antianxiety medication because you are reading this book. If you have a reversible form of depression or anxiety disorder, you will be able to taper off your medication(s) after you have worked on healing your metabolism. This takes time. However, if you are in the middle of a stressful time or are not eating or sleeping well, do not start to taper off your drug just yet. You may need to continue these medications even if you are not depressed or anxious to keep you from self-medicating with alcohol, nicotine, refined sugars and large amounts of caffeine. As long as you are making changes to your habits and are in the process of healing your metabolism, these types of drugs used for a short period of time are not necessarily bad for you.

However, as with all drugs, there are potential side effects when using these medications. Read the package insert carefully. There is a new warning about the increased risk of suicide while on some of these medications so be sure to be monitored appropriately.

Try using a combination of some of the following to help you lower your dose of antidepressants or as a first line therapy for anti-depression: SAM-e, 5 HTP, inositol, L-tyrosine, omega 3 fatty acids, B vitamins, L or D,L phenylalanine and/or acetyl carnitine. For anxiety, try one or more of the following: L-theanine, magnesium, calcium, zinc, taurine, phosphatidyl serine, lecithin, krill oil and/or GABA. If you are interested in natural alternative therapies for mood disorders read *Change Your Brain, Change Your Life* by Daniel Amen, M.D. (Three Rivers Press, 1999).

Other Prescription Drugs

There are many prescription drugs, too numerous to mention here, that cause side effects. If you are taking prescription drugs, discuss with your physician the option of stopping or lowering the dose of any of your medications, or switching to another medicine with fewer side

effects. Be aware that you may be taking a medicine because of another drug's side effects. Be sure you know the reasons you are taking your specific drugs.

Questions to Ask Your Physician and Pharmacist About Your Prescription Medication

1. Why am I taking this medication?
2. Am I taking the lowest dose possible that will still help me with my personal medical issue?
3. Is it time to re-evaluate the need for this drug?
4. Is there anything I can do through diet and other habits to get off this medication?
5. Are there any natural supplements I can use to help me get off my medication?
6. Is there a better medication, one with fewer side effects, that I can be taking?
7. What are the most common side effects of this medication?
8. Do any of my drugs interfere with the action of my other drugs or make me need to use additional drugs?
9. Please show me the data supporting the use of my medication in preventing the risk of a serious medical condition. (For instance, the data showing that the cholesterol lowering medication I am using prevents a heart attack.)

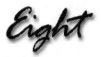

Exercise

The Schwarzbein Way:

A moderate cross-training exercise program that incorporates resistance (adaptive) and flexibility (calming) elements as the main components, with cardiovascular (stimulating) exercises for fun, if at all.

When done correctly, the effect of the right exercise program will help you rebuild lean body tissues and burn off fat weight. The effect of the wrong kind of exercise program breaks down your body and leads to serious health problems—just the thing you were working so hard to avoid.

The most common mistakes regarding exercise are the following:

- Not eating well or sleeping enough to support an exercise program;
- Thinking that the more you exercise the healthier you are;

- Using exercise as a way to self-medicate;
- Believing that cardiovascular exercise is the only kind of exercise that is good for your heart;
- Not doing any resistance exercises;
- Not stretching enough; and
- Not exercising at all.

Exercise for Health

The key to having good health and an ideal body composition is to integrate into your life a moderate exercise routine that will not require escalating amounts of activity to keep you healthy. A moderate exercise program helps you heal or prevent damage to your metabolism, improve your mental function, increase your sense of well-being and achieve the body composition you want. Therefore, the right kind and amount of exercise is important in keeping you healthy, emotionally strong and happy. However, keep in mind that the benefits will not occur if you are overexercising or if you are not eating or sleeping well. If you feel worse after exercising, re-evaluate your program.

Benefits of *Moderate* Exercise

Exercise helps you to . . .
- Boost your energy, your self-esteem and your sense of well-being;
- Achieve your ideal body composition;
- Improve your bowel movements and sleep patterns;
- Retain your independence as you age by maintaining muscle tone and strength;
- Improve coordination and balance decreasing the risk of bone fractures and other injuries;
- Lower your blood pressure and improve heart function;
- Normalize your cholesterol and blood-sugar levels;
- Reduce the risk of the degenerative diseases of aging;
- Usually decrease the cost of your medical care.

Cross-Training Exercise Program

There are three types of activities you could eventually include in any cross-training exercise program: flexibility exercises, resistance training and cardiovascular exercises. For the purpose of metabolic healing, I am going to re-categorize these common types of exercise as calming, adaptive and stimulating. Calming exercises are those where you move or stretch your body with minimal intensity. Adaptive exercises are those that involve spurts of moderate to high intensity with adequate recovery periods and stimulating exercises are those where you continuously work at a moderate to high intensity without sufficient recovery time.

Minimal or low intensity means that you are not breaking a sweat and your heart is not beating faster than 90 beats per minute. You should be able to carry on a conversation easily while doing this type

of exercise. Moderate intensity is when your heart rate is above 90 beats a minute and you huff and puff a bit when trying to talk. High intensity is when you are working at a pace that is difficult to sustain for more than 60 seconds and you find it hard to talk while doing.

In order to be a pure adaptive workout, you need to let your heart rate recover to at or below 90 beats a minute for 60 to 90 seconds every few minutes of exercise. If you do a form of exercise that is a combination of stimulating and adaptive training, consider it a stimulating exercise only.

Calming exercises are good for lowering stress responses in your body, adaptive exercises are good for helping you rebuild lean body tissue and/or burn off fat, and stimulating exercises release feel good chemicals and cause you to break down both lean body tissues and fat. All types of exercise initially can cause positive fat weight loss; however, if you only do stimulating exercises, you will eventually break down too much lean body tissue, damage your metabolism and, ironically, store more fat.

Calming Exercises—Low Intensity

- Stretching exercises
- Restorative yoga
- Tai chi
- *Slow walking—keeping your heart rate below 90 beats per minute at all times
- *Slow swimming—keeping your heart rate below 90 beats per minute at all times

---

*If you are so out of shape that you cannot keep your heart rate below 90 beats a minute, do not count this as a calming exercise.

Adaptive Exercises—Moderate to High Intensity with Rest Periods

- Ball and band work
- Core strength exercises/mat classes/calisthenics
- Light weight routine
- Pilates—Pilates is a full-body exercise program designed by Joseph Pilates in the 1930s that improves strength, flexibility, balance and muscular symmetry
- Pool exercises
- Yoga—strengthening types of yoga only

*Stimulating Exercises—Moderate to High Intensity without Rest Periods

- Aerobic machines such as stair-steppers and exercise bikes
- Aerobics classes
- Bikrum yoga
- Fast biking
- Fast swimming
- Fast walking/hiking
- Kickboxing
- Running/jogging
- Soccer, tennis, volleyball or other vigorous sports
- Spinning exercise bike classes
- Weight lifting-heavy
- Any other stimulating exercises not mentioned

———————

*These could theoretically be considered adaptive exercises if you did them in short bursts of moderate to high intensity and your heart rate recovers at or below 90 beats a minute for one to two minutes every few minutes of exercise.

Exercising Smarter, Not Harder

Most Americans believe that the more cardiovascular or stimulating exercise they do, the longer they will live, the better their heart will function and the more fat they will burn. This could not be more wrong. Consider this fact: on average, a Tibetan monk who does yoga and meditates lives longer and has less heart disease than an American athlete who is involved in some type of running sport.

The truth is that overdoing cardiovascular or stimulating exercises is bad for your heart and your metabolism because it breaks you down, especially after the age of 35 to 40 when you are entering the normal aging phase of your life. The more you do of these types of exercise, the faster you will age and the more heart attacks you can expect, and the only type of weight loss you will "successfully" achieve is the loss of lean body tissues that include organs, bones and muscle. And like any drug (yes, stimulating exercise can be considered a drug) your body becomes conditioned to the stimulation and begins to need more of it to achieve the same results. This means that the more stimulating exercise you do, the more stimulating exercise you will have to do to see the same "benefits". This is analogous to needing to eat less and less when you are on a low calorie intake diet to continue to lose or keep your weight off. In fact, the physiology is the same.

The good news is that stimulating/cardiovascular exercise is not the only type of exercise that is good for your heart. Adaptive exercise also improves cardiovascular performance, without the negative stimulating effect on your metabolism. Therefore, contrary to popular belief, you don't have to do *any* stimulating exercises to keep your heart healthy.

Without doing any stimulating/ cardiovascular exercises ever again, you can still protect your heart and be extremely healthy. You do this by doing adaptive types of exercises.

Exercise Prescription

In general you will be asked to only exercise five times a week, sometimes less. The types and duration of exercise will be determined by your current metabolism. If you have a healthy metabolism you can exercise longer and do stimulating exercises (see Maintenance Plan page 247). If you have a damaged metabolism you need to exercise for less time and are not allowed to do any stimulating exercises (see Healing Plan page 220). No matter how healthy your metabolism, you should not be exercising more than five days a week because you need to give your body time to rebuild. However, all calming exercises can be done every day, if desired.

Getting Medical Clearance

If you are out of shape and over the age of fifty, consult your physician for clearance to exercise. If you have multiple health problems, consider starting your program at an exercise rehabilitation center. Your physician can advise you about facilities in your area. If you have any back, neck or joint problems, *always consult your physician* before starting any exercise routine.

A Simple, Effective Exercise Routine

The following ten exercises are easy, effective and a great way to get you exercising again. They can be done at home in as little as 15 to 20 minutes. The health plans later in this book will give you specific instructions on how and when to do them.

You can mix and match the order of the adaptive and calming exercises to keep your routine more interesting. A good way to do this is to do the calming exercises in between sets of adaptive exercises to

lower your heart rate and maintain good range of motion.

Always start any exercise program with a five-minute warm up to get your muscles warm and loose. This will help avoid injuries. You can walk on a treadmill, march in place or do anything that gets your heart rate up around 100 to 120 beats a minute. Be sure to do this for only 5 minutes. Longer than that and you are starting to do stimulating exercises.

Adaptive: Exercises 1–6

Do 8 to 12 repetitions (one set) of each adaptive exercise. If you want, after resting and getting your heart rate back down for a few minutes, repeat the exercise for a total of two sets.

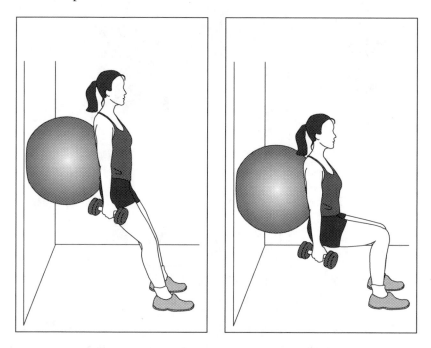

1. **Ball Wall Squat**—Start without the dumbbell weights in your hands. (As you progress and exercise consistently start adding small amounts of weight to make this more difficult.)

> A. Place ball in the small of your back and lean back against it. You should have your feet about six inches away from where they would be if you were standing straight up so you are leaning against the ball.
> B. Sit back and down until you are at a right angle at your knee and hip joints (you may need to reposition your feet to achieve this). If you are a beginner or have knee problems, start by only coming down halfway to 45 degrees.
> C. Stand back up without locking your knees.
> D. Repeat.

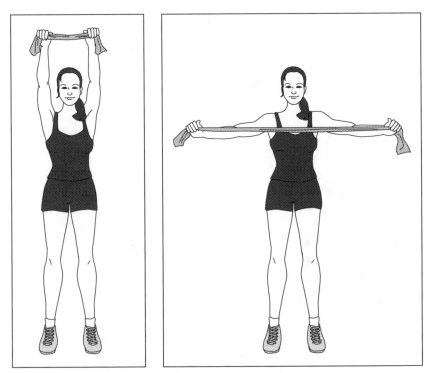

2. **Lat Pull Apart**—Knot band at both ends and grip at knots.

A. Raise straight arms over head.

B. Keeping arms straight, pull arms open and down so that you finish with band touching chest and pulled apart as far as possible with arms open wide at shoulder level. If this isn't difficult enough, move your hands closer together on the band.

C. Raise your arms above your head again. Be sure to not snap or bounce band on the way back up.

D. Repeat.

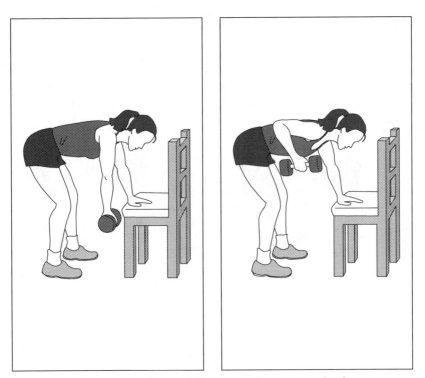

3. **One Arm Row**—Start with one to three pounds if you are new to lifting weights.

A. Place hands on a chair in front of you, extend spine to create a table-top with your back. Take one hand off the chair and slide other hand over to the middle. With free hand, grab dumbbell.

B. Bring elbow straight up to ceiling and turn your wrist clockwise so the dumbbell ends up tucked sideways against your body at chest level.

C. Reverse the motion and slowly bring the dumbell back down to the starting position.

D. Repeat.

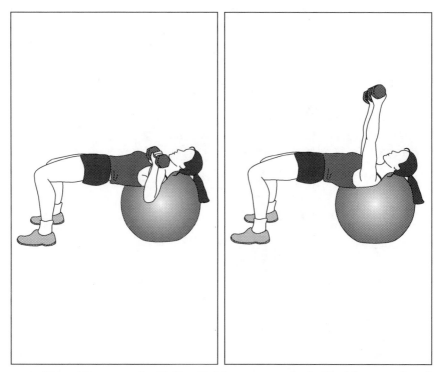

4. **Chest Press on the Ball**—Bridge out on the ball with your shoulder blades resting in the center of the ball and your head and neck supported. Keep your hips up by contracting your buttocks and spinal muscles throughout the set. Start with your hands at your shoulders.

> A. Push the dumbbells up and together over your chest so the weights meet in the middle when your arms are fully extended.
>
> B. Bring the dumbbells back down, following the same pattern in reverse.
>
> C. Repeat

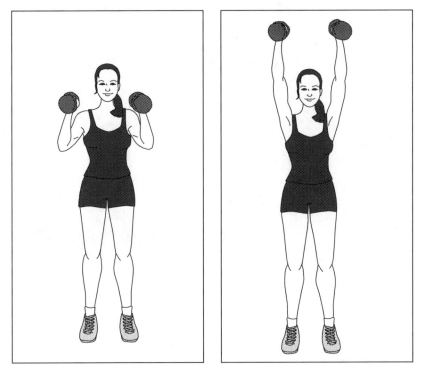

5. **Overhead Press**—Stand with your feet shoulder-width apart, knees slightly bent, and pull bellybutton into the spine (start with 1 to 3 pound weights).

A. Start with hands at shoulders, and thumbs pointing towards shoulders.

B. Raise dumbbells straight up toward the ceiling, keeping hands slightly in front of shoulders so that when you finish you can see your hands in your peripheral vision.

C. Bring the dumbbells slowly back down to the starting position.

D. Repeat.

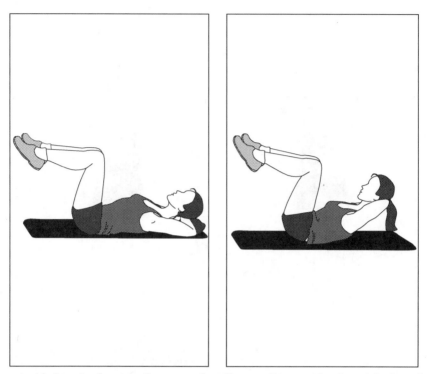

6. **Abdominal crunches on the floor**—Lie on back with hands behind neck and knees bent, feet off the floor. Pretend there is a grapefruit between your chin and your chest as you perform the movement.

A. Lift up from your shoulder blades and your tailbone, bringing your head, arms and shoulders, and hips off the ground. Make sure the small of your back stays in contact with the floor.

B. Slowly bring your head and hips back to the beginning position.

C. Repeat.

Calming Exercises: 7–10

Hold each stretch for at least 30 seconds on each side. Repeat one more time on each side for a more complete stretch.

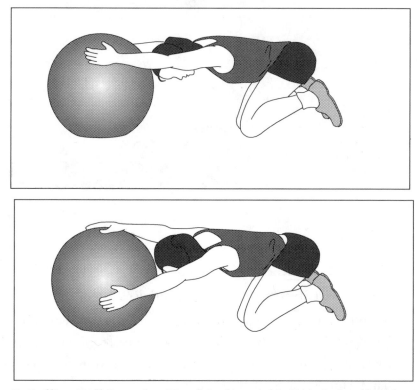

7. **Rolling Ball Stretch**—Kneel in front of ball and place hands on the top of the ball, shoulder-width apart with arms extended. Sit back slightly towards heels.

    A. Roll ball towards one side and hold for at least 30 seconds.

    B. Repeat to other side.

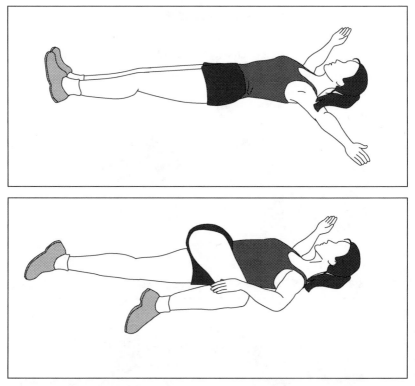

8. **Spinal Twist Stretch**—Lie on back with legs extended.

A. Pull right knee to chest and take left hand on outside of right knee and pull towards left side of floor while reaching away with right arm, palm up. Turn your head to look at your outstretched hand. Hold for at least 30 seconds.

B. Repeat to other side.

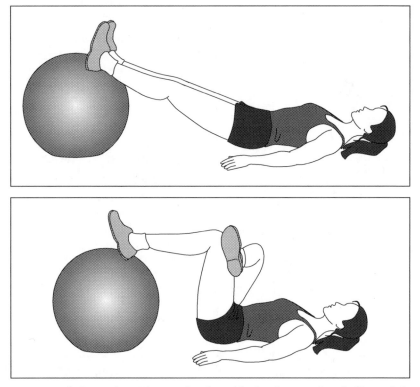

9. **Pretzel Stretch**—Lie on back with heels on the ball and legs extended.

A. Keeping hips on the ground, put right ankle just above left knee and roll ball in, bending left knee and stretching the buttock/hip area on the right side. Hold for at least 30 seconds.

B. For a deeper stretch, use the same side hand and gently push your knee away from your body.

C. Repeat to the other side.

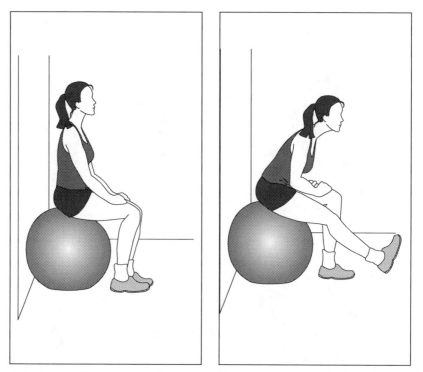

10. **Seated Hamstring Stretch**—Sit on ball. Extend right leg with foot flexed.

A. Put hands on left thigh, lift chest and keep your back extended as you lean forward. Hold for at least 30 seconds.

B. Then point your toes and hold stretch for another 30 seconds.

C. Repeat to other side.

Helpful Exercise Tips

In order to have a good workout, follow these helpful tips:

- Get plenty of sleep every night to avoid injuries.
- Drink plenty of water to keep hydrated.
- Stretch for 15 minutes at the end of your exercise routine.
- Remember to breathe. Your breathing should be regular and deep—from the abdominal area. You should breathe out during the strenuous part of your exercise—such as lifting a weight or hitting a tennis ball—and breathe in during the recovery phase.
- Eat well. Do not lower your caloric intake, eliminate food groups or skip meals. If you exercise and do not eat, your body will break down more than rebuild.
- The best time to exercise is whenever you can.
- Vary your exercise routine to keep it interesting and avoid overuse injuries.
- Keep your workout schedule the same to ensure consistency. Treat it as you would an important appointment.
- Work out with friends or a personal trainer if you have a hard time keeping to a schedule.
- Make sure you have the proper shoes and equipment for the activity you have chosen.
- Be consistent and have fun!

Nine

Hormones

The Schwarzbein Way:

Use hormone replacement therapy when needed to replace any hormone your body can't produce enough of naturally, using a bioidentical hormone taken to mimic your body's normal production and secretion of the hormone being replaced.

The first four steps of the Schwarzbein Principle Program are designed to heal your metabolism or keep it healthy by balancing the hormone systems of your body. This works as long as they are still functioning. However, if you no longer produce a hormone, you will not be able to balance your system completely without Step 5—Hormone Replacement Therapy (HRT), as needed. Without full balance, you will not be able to heal and you will age faster and be less healthy.

If you are still having problems or don't feel revitalized, energetic, and better than you've ever felt in your life after completing the first

four steps in this program, you may have a hormone problem. If you already know or suspect that you have a hormone problem before starting this program, get tested and start hormone replacement therapy before working on Steps 3 and 4. Ideally, you will be working on fixing your hormone problems at the same time that you are working on Steps 1 and 2.

The most common mistakes regarding HRT are the following:

• Taking a drug hormone instead of a bioidentical hormone;
• Taking a hormone incorrectly;
• Taking a hormone that your body can still make;
• Not monitoring the effects of the hormone you are taking with frequent lab work and appropriate studies; and
• Not taking a hormone that is missing.

You can have a hormone deficiency state whether you have a healthy or a damaged metabolism. If you have a healthy metabolism, you can take the exact dose of the hormone right away and your problems should clear up quickly. If you have a damaged metabolism, balancing the missing hormone is harder than you might think and requires starting with small doses and making small adjustments over a longer period of time. This can be difficult to achieve, and you will probably need to be treated by a hormone specialist and not your primary care physician in order to accomplish this task. Don't be put off by the effort and time it will take to do this step right. A low or nonexistent hormone may be the reason that your health is not improving despite working on your other habits. In that instance, Step 5 becomes as important as all the other steps combined.

If you feel that you may have a hormone problem keeping you from health or healing, you need to have your hormone levels checked. It is essential to make the diagnosis of a low hormone state before you start taking hormone replacement therapy.

Four Simple Rules for Hormone Replacement Therapy

When taking a prescribed hormone to replace a hormone that the body can no longer make, it is important to understand that certain rules need to be followed in order to achieve true balance. If you follow my four simple rules for hormone replacement therapy, it is hard to go wrong.

- **Identify the hormone(s) that needs to be replaced.** Although you do not have to wait for a hormone to be completely gone before starting to replace it, do not replace a hormone that can still be produced appropriately. Laboratory work is the best way to identify missing hormones. Unfortunately, not all labs can run hormone levels accurately; therefore, your blood or saliva samples need to be run through specific labs. (check out my Web site for specific recommendations at *www.schwarzbeinprinciple.com*)

- **Replace the missing hormone with the same (identical) hormone.** This is common sense but it is not followed all the time. The most accurate terminology for taking the same hormone is "bioidentical" hormone replacement therapy.

- **Mimic normal physiology as much as possible.** Take the hormone how and when the body used to produce and secrete it throughout the day or month. This is another very common-sense approach that is not always being followed.

- **Take HRT seriously and monitor it appropriately.** This means following the hormone effects through hormone levels, how you feel, and making sure that the positive changes that should be occurring are happening and conversely that unwanted side effects, are not occurring.

HRT, If Needed

It is extremely important to replace a hormone if it is missing. If you have a healthy metabolism, fixing your hormone problem will help your other hormones get balanced immediately. If you have a damaged metabolism, HRT, if needed, becomes one more important step in getting you to feel and be better.

Here are some common hormone imbalances that are discussed in this chapter:

- Hypothyroid/low thyroid
- Low insulin or high insulin
- Adrenal gland burnout
- Progesterone issues
- Estradiol issues
- Testosterone issues

In each section below, I list the most common symptoms associated with each of the hormone problems and what tests need to be ordered to determine the missing or out of balance hormone(s). Make sure to have your levels tested when you are not sick or taking drugs on a short-term basis that can affect your hormone levels. This will decrease the chance of you being misdiagnosed with a hormone problem when you don't really have one. Mimicking normal physiology and tracking is more complicated and will be left up to your treating physician. However, I will provide some pearls of wisdom to help you get into better balance.

If you have multiple hormone issues and are having problems with your health, I highly recommend that you work with a reputable endocrinologist or a physician who specilizes in hormones who can help you balance your missing hormones. The balancing of several hormone systems at once is complicated because of the interaction between all hormone systems. In general you need to adjust all

hormone systems if one needs adjustment. For example, if you are taking both thyroid hormone and estradiol replacement therapy and your thyroid dose needs adjusting, it is very likely that you will have to adjust your estradiol doses, too.

Note: Just because you have the symptoms of a hormone problem does not mean you have that problem. You need to be tested and treated by a professional. Do not try to correct hormone problems yourself by taking over-the-counter or non-prescription hormone preparations.

Hypothyroid or Low Thyroid

The following advice is for garden-variety low thyroid disease (hypothyroidism), not for rare pituitary disorders that cause low thyroid problems. If you have one of these rare problems, you *must* be seen by an endocrinologist.

Common Symptoms of Hypothyroidism:
- Achy muscles
- Approximately 10-pound weight gain or the inability to lose weight
- Cold intolerance
- Constipation
- Dry skin
- Fatigue
- Hair loss
- Headaches
- Low mood
- Lower body temperature
- PMS and irregular cycles or heavier menstrual bleeding
- Sleep problems (sleeping too much or not able to sleep enough)

The Test: ———————————————————————

Have your TSH, free T4 and TPO blood serum levels measured. A T3U or T3 uptake level is not a thyroid hormone level. It is a test used to calculate your free T4 level and should not be measured. Make sure you have your free T4 level measured directly, not calculated. T3 hormone levels are not needed to make a diagnosis of hypothyroid disease.

Results: ———————————————————————

- A very high TSH level with or without a low T4 level guarantees you have real thyroid disease.
- If you have an elevated *TPO antibody, you have an active autoimmune problem. If it is negative, you probably don't have an autoimmune process or it is no longer active.
- If you have the symptoms but do not have the hormone levels to back up the diagnosis, you probably have a hormone problem but not a thyroid hormone problem. Have your cortisol and DHEA and/or insulin levels checked to rule out adrenal gland burnout or insulin resistance.

——————

If you have a positive TPO with or without obvious low thyroid problems, consider that you may have a problem with your gastrointestinal tract and get evaluated. See my Web site, www.schwarzbeinprinciple.com for further information.

The Correct (identical) Hormone: ———————————————

- The bioidentical equivalent replacement for T4 is levothyroxine.
- The bioidentical equivalent replacement for T3 is liothyronine.

There are many good preparations available through prescription for both of these.

Dosage and Scheduling: ———————————————————

- Normally you only have to take one dose of T4 in the morning to mimic normal.
- If you have had thyroid disease for a long time, have had your

thyroid removed or ablated with radioactive iodine, you may need a separate low dose T3 prescription as well as your T4 prescription. This is determined by checking your T3 levels after you have started T4 therapy.

- Most people will *not* have to take thyroid hormone on an empty stomach as advocated in the literature. This is one of the easiest hormones to replace. You should replace it around your habits, not change your habits to accommodate your thyroid pill. However, don't take your thyroid pill with iron. If you are one of the few people who do not absorb thyroid well, you will have to take it on an empty stomach.
- Never use a fixed ratio combination pill of T4 and T3. This includes glandulars and any thyroid preparation that comes in grains such as Armour. Also you should never take a T3 preparation without T4. If you are taking any of these preparations or T3 alone to treat low thyroid disease, you probably are not mimicking normal physiology.

Monitoring: —————————————————————

- Follow TSH and free T4 levels
- Follow T3 levels, too, if you are also taking a T3 prescription or to determine if you need to.
- You do not need to follow TPO levels to determine the dose of your thyroid medication.
- The most important goal is to get your TSH level around one to two. Secondly, if you are taking T3, try to keep T3 levels from being much higher than T4 levels.
- Do not check TSH levels sooner than every six weeks. If you check your levels too soon, you can be making changes that are inappropriate.
- If your TSH levels are below normal, you are taking too much thyroid hormone and you need to lower your dose(s); if your TSH is above normal, you are not taking enough thyroid hormone

replacement therapy and you will need to increase your doses.

- It is important to make small adjustments in thyroid doses. Increasing by 12 to 25 microgram increments is highly recommended for T4 and by 2.5 microgram increments for T3.
- Once your thyroid levels are stable, have your TSH checked every six months and a T4, T3 and TSH level every year.
- If all your symptoms are due to low thyroid, they will all completely go away once your hormone levels are normal. If you are still having symptoms, look for another cause and don't keep taking higher and higher doses of thyroid medication.

If you are taking too much thyroid hormone replacement, you can end up with the following problems:

- Anxiety
- Bone loss or full blown osteoporosis
- Decreased memory and concentration
- Excessive sweating
- Fatigue
- Hair loss
- Heat intolerance including hot flashes and night sweats
- Irregular heart beats or arrythmias
- Irregular menstrual cycles (women)
- Lean body tissue weight loss
- Peeling finger nails
- Rapid heart beats or palpitations
- Sleep disturbances—hard time falling or staying asleep
- Weakness
- Weight gain (yes, too much thyroid hormone therapy can cause weight gain by destroying lean body tissue and worsening your metabolism)

Insulin

Low insulin levels can be due to diabetes (pancreatic failure) or to malnourishment from not eating enough food or enough carbohydrates and overexercising. High insulin levels can be due to stress, overeating, low estradiol, chronic yo-yo dieting, smoking tobacco and/or drinking alcohol. In either case you want to know your insulin levels to determine if you need to replace insulin or work on habits that normalize insulin levels.

Anyone who has high blood sugar levels should have their insulin levels checked at least once to determine if they have Type I (insulin deficient) or Type II (insulin resistant) diabetes. If you have diabetes, I highly recommend that you work with a reputable diabetes specialist. This includes internists and family practitioners who have made diabetes part of their specialty.

Common Symptoms of Low Insulin Levels:

- Excessive urination
- Dizziness
- Fatigue
- Fruity breath
- Fuzzy brain
- Increased hunger or thirst
- Irregular menstrual cycles
- Irritability
- Low mood
- Muscle weakness and/or achiness
- Poor memory or concentration
- Poor wound healing, skin funguses or vaginal yeast infections
- Sleep disturbances
- Sugar cravings
- Unexpected or very easy weight loss

Common Symptoms of High Insulin Levels:

- Acne
- Ankle swelling
- Burning feet
- Constipation
- Decreased memory or concentration
- Depression
- Fatigue
- Fluctuating high blood pressure readings
- Fuzzy brain
- Irregular menstrual cycles and/or anovulatory cycles
- Irritability
- Loose bowel movements alternating with constipation
- Sugar cravings
- Water retention
- Weight gain especially around the middle

The Tests:

You determine your insulin status by measuring insulin levels using fasting blood samples run at a laboratory that specializes in endocrine tests along with fasting blood sugar and triglyceride levels.

Results:

- Very low insulin levels and very high blood sugar levels associated with weight loss, fatigue and excessive thirst and urination guarantees, with a few exceptions, the diagnosis of Type I diabetes (insulin deficient diabetes). You must use insulin replacement therapy to prevent death and to get healthy.
- If you have type II diabetes (insulin resistant diabetes) and your fasting insulin level is low or in the normal range when your blood sugar or triglyceride levels are high, you qualify for

short-term insulin therapy. It is imporant to take insulin at this stage of Type II diabetes because your pancreas is failing to produce enough insulin to treat your high blood sugar and triglyceride levels. Left untreated this will lead to full failure of the pancreas and the need for lifelong insulin. However, if your insulin levels are very high, you can work on your lifestyle habits to help lower them back down. Refer back to steps 1 through 4.

• If you have normal blood sugar levels, high triglyceride levels and high insulin levels, you are insulin resistant. There is no need for insulin therapy at this stage. Work on your nutrition and lifestyle habits (steps 1 through 4) to help you become insulin sensitive again.

• If you have low insulin levels with normal blood sugar levels and low to normal triglyceride levels, you are not eating enough food and/or enough carbohydrates for your daily activities. You are not building efficiently and will need to reevaluate your nutrition and exercise habits and adjust them appropriately.

The Correct (identical) Hormone: ————————————

• The bioidentical form of insulin is . . . insulin.

• There are now "designer" insulin's that are very similar to the insulin made in the pancreas. These types of insulin are being prescribed more frequently because they either act faster and are eliminated more rapidly (short acting) or they do not peak at all (long-acting) and, therefore, improve sugar control without as many low blood sugar reactions and without keeping high levels of insulin around in the blood stream for long periods of time. Although they are not 100 percent identical, they are close enough and so far seem to be beneficial without adverse side effects.

Dosage and Scheduling: ————————————————

• You need multiple doses of insulin throughout the day to mimic the normal functioning of the pancreas. This can be accomplished

with the insulin pump or with a combination of long and short acting insulin injections.

- If you have Type II diabetes you may only need a long acting insulin once a day or small amounts of short acting insulin before meals. You rarely need full insulin replacement. An exception is someone with advanced stage Type II diabetes with full blown pancreatic failure.

Monitoring:

Type I Diabetes:

- You track insulin therapy for Type I diabetes by tracking your blood sugar levels through home finger-stick blood sugar monitoring throughout the day. The goal is to have lower blood sugar levels before meals and slightly higher after meals. Before meal ranges of 60 to 140 are acceptable. You can even be slightly lower as long as you do not get hypoglycemic reactions. After meals, you want to aim for levels of 160 or less. Work with your endocrinologist or internist to come up with ranges that are specific for you as these are first target blood sugar ranges and more tight control needs to be achieved over time.

- Your initial goal is to achieve a HbA1C level of 7 percent or less. HbA1C is an estimation of the three-month average of your blood sugar levels. This test needs to be done every three to six months to determine treatment changes (including lifestyle habits). Once you reached that first target, you want to shoot for normal range HbA1C levels without episodes of low blood sugar reactions.

- At the same time, you want to make sure that your cholesterol levels normalize or stay normal with your insulin therapy and that you monitor your eyes, kidneys and peripheral nerves for damage due to high blood sugar levels.

- You cannot just take all the insulin you want. Initially, too much

insulin causes low blood sugar reactions and fat weight gain. Over time too much insulin increases your risk for cancer, cholesterol problems, gout, heart attacks, high blood pressure disease, Stein-Leventhal syndrome, and strokes. However, not enough insulin means that you will not be able to rebuild your body chemicals on a daily basis. This causes accelerated aging and is more harmful than too much insulin.

- If you have Type I diabetes, a good approximation of the amount of insulin you require in a day is 0.6 units of insulin for every kilogram of body weight (weight in pounds divided by 2.2 = weight in kilograms). If you are not taking enough insulin because you are starving yourself to stay thin, or not eating enough carbohydrates because you think that they are bad for you, you need to increase your insulin and balance out your nutrition. If you are taking much more than this amount of insulin each day, you need to improve your nutrition and lifestyle habits. That's where the first four steps of my Program come in.

Type II Diabetes:

- You monitor insulin therapy and/or the response to changing your nutrition and lifestyle habits by tracking your blood sugar levels before and after meals. The first goal is to achieve a blood sugar level at any time of the day that is less than or equal to *160. Do not try and reach this goal immediately. Most of you will not be able to achieve these numbers without starving yourself or overexercising. That is why it is so important to work with a diabetes specialist. If you starve yourself to reach this goal, you will never heal.

- If you have Type II diabetes and are taking more than 1 unit of insulin per kilogram of body weight, you are probably on too

---

Please note that the first response to lowering blood sugar levels if you have Type II diabetes is usually an increase in triglyceride and cholesterol levels. This is a normal response and should not be treated with statin drugs. However, you can use the newer insulin sensitizing drugs to help lower your cholesterol and/or triglyceride levels, if they continue to stay elevated.

much insulin. You may need to add in some of the newer insulin sensitizing drugs (discuss what these are with your diabetes specialist) or change the dose of drugs you are already taking. You will also need to make changes to your nutrition and lifestyle habits. That's where the first four steps of my Program come in.

Insulin Resistance:

• You monitor insulin and triglyceride levels to track the response to the treatment of insulin resistance. The goal is to lower insulin levels back to normal but only after triglyceride levels have come back down. You need to make sure that you are not starving yourself or overexercising to lower your insulin levels. You will only be able to completely reverse insulin resistance if you understand that you need to heal your metabolism first. You may require one of the newer insulin sensitizing drugs (ask your internist or endocrinologist) in order to help you become insulin sensitive again. Consider taking one of them if you have dug yourself into a deep metabolic hole and the first 4 steps of my program do not make a dent in any of your blood levels after 3 to 6 months.

Cortisol and DHEA

The symptoms of cortisol and dehydroepiandrosterone (DHEA) problems overlap the symptoms of thyroid and insulin problems. If you do not have either of these conditions, but continue to have symptoms, you should have your cortisol and DHEA levels checked. The recommendations below pertain to adrenal gland burnout only and not to Addison's disease*.

Addison's disease, an autoimmune destruction of your adrenal glands, is a much more serious condition than adrenal gland burnout that requires very precise replacement therapy. If you have Addison's disease, consult your endocrinologist for your hormone replacement needs.

Common Symptoms of Adrenal Gland Burnout:

- Allergies
- Anxiety or depression
- Asthma
- Cold intolerance
- Constipation
- Depression
- Digestive problems such as intestinal bloating and feeling like you are not digesting your food
- Dizziness
- Fatigue—from mild to debilitating
- Headaches
- Inability to lose weight
- Irritability
- Irritable bowel syndrome
- Low blood pressure
- Severe PMS
- Sleep disruption
- Or you have "classic" symptoms of either low thyroid or insulin resistance but your thyroid and insulin levels are normal,

The Tests: ————————————————————

Cortisol levels are checked by adrenal saliva testing (not blood testing) at a reputable lab such as Diagnostechs Inc., BioHealth Diagnostechs and Great Smokies Lab. There are many medications that interfere with this test. Make sure that you ask the physician who ordered this test if any prescription or over-the-counter medications you are taking interfere with your levels.

DHEA levels are checked by either DHEA saliva tests or blood levels of DHEA sulfate.

Results:

When interpreting adrenal saliva testing, it is important to know what you did on the day of collection as well as your pre-existing habits. Your health care provider must use all this information to determine what stage you are in because he/she will have to take into account what your levels should have been for what you are doing relative to your test results. For example, if you are skipping meals and exercising you should have very high cortisol and DHEA levels. If they come back within the normal ranges, you are probably in late stage 2 or early stage 3 of adrenal gland burnout (see below).

In general, if you have adrenal gland burnout, it is better to change your lifestyle habits first before taking hormone replacement therapy. By taking hormones, you may make yourself feel better for the moment but if you maintain the same bad habits that led you to burn out in the first place, you will never heal.

There are three major stages of adrenal gland burnout:

- Stage 1 (early)—both DHEA levels and cortisol levels are very high. Or cortisol levels are very high but DHEA levels are normal. Never take cortisol in this stage. However, if your DHEA levels are normal, you can use small amounts of DHEA for a short period of time to balance out the higher cortisol levels until the stress causing the high cortisol levels is fixed. This does not mean that it is okay to take DHEA for an extended period of time because you are not working on changing your habits!
- Stage 2 (intermediate)—DHEA and cortisol levels are mismatched (one is higher than the other) within the normal to low ranges. You may consider taking cortisol replacement therapy but it is best to work on lifestyle habits in this stage. Or if your DHEA level is very low, you can try small amounts of DHEA to help balance out the cortisol to DHEA ratio.
- Stage 3 (advanced)—both DHEA and cortisol levels are too low.

If you cannot function and you cannot afford to stay in bed and rest until you are healed, you can take appropriate amounts of both hormones in this stage.

The Correct (identical) Hormone: ————————————————

- Hydrocortisone and cortisol are both used to replace cortisol.
- DHEA is the hormone used to replace itself.
- Pregnenolone is a hormone that can be converted into cortisol and DHEA in your body. You can use pregnenolone to help your body make more of either. Take with biotin to help convert more pregnenolone to cortisol.
- Prednisone should not be used for hormone replacement therapy. It is a cortisone-like drug that is used for inflammatory conditions such as asthma, skin allergies and autoimmune diseases.
- Do not take adrenal glandulars unless they just have cortisol in them in a known quantity. In general, glandulars are not standardized; therefore, you don't know what else is in them or at what dose you are getting cortisol/cortisone.

Dosage and Scheduling: ————————————————

- There is a changing pattern of cortisol in your body throughout the day and night. You start to secrete much higher levels of cortisol starting at 3 A.M., which peak around 7 to 10 A.M., then taper down until 3 P.M. After 3 P.M. the levels become slightly lower and stay low the rest of the afternoon and night. Therefore, the bulk of your hydrocortisone/cortisol dose should be taken in the morning with a slightly smaller dose taken at 3 to 4 P.M. Taking hydrocortisone/cortisol too late in the day can keep you from sleeping well.
- You can also use very small amounts of hydrocortisone/cortisol at the times in the day that your testing shows you to be the most deficient.
- You can take higher doses of pregnenolone once a day in the

morning instead of hydrocortisone/cortisol to see if your body will produce more cortisol from it. Take with biotin to avoid the pregnenolone converting to DHEA. You can try this at any time in either stage 2 or 3 but never in stage 1.

• DHEA secretion is more consistent throughout a 24-hour time period; therefore, you can take the same amount of DHEA twice a day. Men need higher amounts of DHEA (average 25mg to 100mg a day). Women require much less (average 2.5mg to 20mg a day).

Monitoring: _____

• If you are taking higher doses of hydrocortisone or cortisol, do not follow saliva cortisol levels because they are no longer accurate. You will need to monitor blood cortisol and ACTH levels. If your ACTH levels go too low, you know you are taking too much cortisone or cortisol.

• If you are taking small amounts of cortisol (1 to 3 mg at a time), you can still follow with salivary testing. Adjust the amount you take to achieve mid normal to high normal cortisol levels.

• Follow DHEA levels by either testing salivary DHEA levels or blood DHEA sulfate levels (DHEA-S).

• DHEA is an androgen and will block the action of estrogens. Monitor estradiol effect when taking DHEA.

• If you are on pregnenolone, follow pregnenolone blood levels and both cortisol and DHEA salivary levels.

In general, I have found that both peri-menopausal and menopausal women have the hardest time adjusting to DHEA and sometimes even pregnenolone replacement therapy. It is still worth trying them if DHEA or cortisol levels are very low. However, because they both can block the action of estrogen, you need to monitor carefully for anti-estrogen side effects ranging from irritability, hair loss, abnormal hair growth, weight gain around the midsection and acne to hot flashes, vaginal dryness, decreased libido and disrupted sleep.

If you are taking too much cortisol you can end up with the following problems:

- Anxiety
- Bone loss
- Decreased memory and/or concentration
- Depression
- Easy bruising
- Fat weight around your midsection
- Hair loss or thinning
- Higher blood pressure
- Increased carbohydrate cravings
- Irregular periods
- Red rash on your cheeks from broken blood vessels
- Sleep disruptions
- Sodium and potassium electrolyte imbalances
- Thinning of your skin
- Weakness

If you are taking too much DHEA, some of the signs and symptoms are:

- Acne
- Anxiety
- Carbohydrate craving
- Hair loss or thinning
- Increased fat weight around your midsection
- Irritability
- Sleep disruption
- Symptoms of menopause

Progesterone

The term estrogen dominance can be used to describe the situation when the body has too much total estrogen for the amount of progesterone. It never means that you should take progesterone daily

and it doesn't mean you should use progesterone without estrogen (if estrogens are low). If you are truly estrogen dominant and your progesterone levels are low, you should take progesterone replacement therapy to rebalance the system but only for the last 14 days of each menstrual cycle. If progesterone levels are normal, it is time to improve your nutrition and lifestyle habits to help balance out the ratio between estrogens and progestogens; for example, decreasing the over-consumption of alcohol and/or the soy products you are using.

Check your progesterone levels if you have any of the symptoms below, if you want/need to know if you are still ovulating or before starting progesterone therapy.

Common Symptoms of Low Progesterone:

- *Acne
- Arthritic-like pains
- *Breast tenderness and/or enlargement
- Decreased memory and/or concentration
- Decreased sex drive
- *Depression/irritability
- Dry skin
- Fatigue
- Hair loss
- Headaches
- *High blood pressure
- *Hot flashes/night sweats
- *Irregular or excessive uterine bleeding, especially with increased clots—may also be caused by nonhormonal problems such as fibroids, adenomyosis or polyps
- Mood swings
- *PMS

- Vaginal dryness
- *Water retention
- *Weight gain around the midsection

*These symptoms are not due to low progesterone per se, but are commonly due to an imbalance between progesterone and estradiol that can occur both naturally and during the adjustment phases of initiating cycling hormone replacement therapy in menopause. Please note that the symptoms of low progesterone completely overlap those of high progesterone so you cannot make a diagnosis of low progesterone without first checking your progesterone levels.

The Tests:

Test your progesterone levels through blood work, *not saliva,* using a reputable lab.

- Check progesterone levels seven days before your menstrual period is due to determine if you are ovulating or need to take progesterone the second half of your cycle.
- Check your progesterone levels two different times, two weeks apart, if your menstrual cycles are so irregular that you cannot reliably determine the seven days before your period is due.
- Check progesterone levels at any time if you are in menopause.

Results:

If your progesterone level is low (use the luteal phase normal ranges found on the lab report to determine this), you qualify for progesterone therapy.

The Correct (identical) Hormone:

- Progesterone is bioidentical for progesterone.
- Prometrium is a noncompounded formula of bioidentical progesterone

that comes in 100mg or 200mg doses. Do not use if you are allergic to peanuts.

• I don't like progesterone topical creams or gels for hormone replacement therapy in menopausal women. They have erratic absorption and noncompliance issues as with any topical hormone therapy. There is also evidence to suggest that topical progesterone does not protect the uterus from abnormal thickening (hyperplasia) and/or cancer because progesterone gets converted in the skin to a form of progesterone (metabolite) that does not work at the uterine level. If you want to bypass your liver, use a compounded sublingual (under the tongue) preparation.

• Provera, aka medroxyprogesterone acetate, is not progesterone— stay away from this drug. Same for Aygestin (norethindrone acetate) or any other synthetic progestin. Ask your pharmacist if what you are taking is pure progesterone.

• The new combipatches do not have bioidentical progesterone in them and don't let anyone tell you that they do!

Dosage and Scheduling: ——————————————————————————

• Progesterone is secreted at much higher levels during the 14 days before your period is due (the luteal phase) and much lower levels during the first 14 days of the cycle (from your period to ovulation or follicular phase). Therefore, you should not take high dose progesterone replacement more than 14 days out of every menstrual month.

• If you have a uterus, cycle with a starting dose of 75mg to 100mg of a sustanined release progesterone pill twice a day, 11 to 14 days of the menstrual cycle. For example start taking progesterone anywhere from cycle days 15 to 18 and finish on day 28 if you are trying to mimic a 28 day cycle.

• If you are in menopause, you may choose to use the calendar month versus the menstrual cycle month and choose to take your

added progesterone twice a day, calendar days 1 through 14. With this option you must take the full 14 days.

- If you don't have a uterus, you can still cycle progesterone 11 to 14 days, whether you are in menopause or just not ovulating. This is a judgment call and will depend on how you are feeling.

- If you are in menopause (no uterus), you can elect to only use smaller doses of progesterone twice a day every day to mimic the normal follicular phase of the menstrual cycle. You would only need to do this if your progesterone level before starting progesterone therapy was too low (use the normal follicular blood ranges to determine this). Start with doses at 0.125mg to 0.25mg of a sublingual prepartion twice a day. This can only be achieved with compounding progesterone since noncompounded formulas have too much progesterone to mimic the small amounts of daily progesterone needed.

Monitoring: ————————————————————————————————

- Progesterone is a stimulant and an estrogen blocker. Taking too much progesterone can initially make you feel better so don't track progesterone based solely on how you feel. Check fasting blood levels of progesterone (do not take your morning dose until after your test) and aim for low normal to mid normal luteal phase ranges. (These are different at each lab so check the ranges provided with your results.) Adjust your progesterone up or down as needed.

- Unlike popular belief you can get too much progesterone. If you are taking too much progesterone, you may have some of the symptoms listed below. Remember that these symptoms can appear years after being on progesterone therapy and may still be related to too much progesterone. Also know that you can have low progesterone levels and still be taking too much progesterone due to not taking enough or having enough estradiol in your body to help balance the progesterone effects.

Note: The symptoms of a high progesterone effect are similar to those of a low progesterone effect and to high and low estradiol effects, too. That is why it is so important that you don't go by how you feel when you replace sex hormones. Have your levels checked through a good lab that specializes in endocrine tests. That is the only way to assure that the blood work results you obtain are accurate.

High Progesterone Effect Causes These Symptoms and Other Problems:

• Acne
• Anxiety
• Bone loss
• Breast tenderness and/or enlargement
• Decreased memory and/or concentration
• Decreased sex drive
• Depression
• Dry skin
• Fatigue
• Hair loss or thinning hair
• Higher blood pressure
• High insulin levels
• Hot flashes
• Irregular to no menses
• Irritability
• Itching
• Joint aches and pains
• Mood swings
• Night sweats
• Rise in total cholesterol, triglyceride and/or LDL cholesterol levels and/or a decrease in HDL cholesterol levels
• Sleep disruptions
• Vaginal dryness
• Weight gain around the midsection

A Chronic High Progesterone Effect Is Associated with the Following Diseases:

- Adrenal gland burnout
- Alzheimer's disease
- Autoimmune disorders
- Breast cancer
- Chronic Insomnia
- Gout
- Heart disease/heart attack/strokes
- High blood pressure
- High triglycerides, high LDL levels and/or low HDL levels
- Metabolic syndrome
- Osteoporosis
- Severe depression
- Type II diabetes

Estradiol

Women have the potential to be at their healthiest when they have peak levels of all hormones. That is why it is important to replace any and all hormones when they are low or missing. Estradiol is no exception. Never ever take progesterone therapy if you do not have enough estradiol to support it. Progesterone blocks the effect of estradiol and will increase the risk of degenerative diseases if taken without enough estradiol to balance it out.

If you want to determine if you are in menopause, need to know if you have enough estradiol to support your progesterone replacement therapy or need to evaluate why your menstrual periods are irregular, lighter or have stopped without a good explanation have your estradiol levels checked.

Common Symptoms and Problems of a Low Estradiol Effect:

- Acne
- Anxiety
- Bone loss
- Breast tenderness and/or enlargement
- Decreased memory and/or concentration
- Decreased sex drive
- Depression
- Dry skin
- Fatigue
- Hair loss or thinning hair
- Higher blood pressure
- Hot flashes
- Irregular to no menses
- Irritability
- Itching
- Joint aches and pains
- Mood swings
- Night sweats
- Sleep disruptions
- Vaginal dryness
- Weight gain around the midsection

The Tests: ————————————————————————————————————

Have your estradiol and FSH levels measured. Estradiol is the human estrogen made in the ovaries; FSH is the pituitary hormone that regulates estradiol production.

Results: ——————————————————————————————————————

- If your estradiol level is low and your FSH level is high you are in menopause and qualify for HRT.

- If your estradiol level is low and your FSH is normal, you are not in *menopause. The most common causes of these results are being underweight, malnourishment, overexercising, birth control pills, drug interactions and stressful conditions. Rarely, this can be a sign of a pituitary tumor.

The Correct (identical) Hormone: ─────────────────────

- Estradiol is the bioidentical hormone used for replacement therapy of an estradiol deficiency state. Do not confuse it with equinol, conjugated estrogens, esterified estrogens, estropipate, or other synthetic estrogens. There are many estradiol preparations available at your local pharmacy from pills to patches such as Estrace, Gynodiol and generic estradiol pills to Vivelle Dot, Alora and Climara patches. Ask your pharmacist for other names of estradiol preparations. Make sure to tell the pharmacist you are looking for estradiol and nothing else since now some of these estradiol products are being combined with nonbioidentical progestins.
- The best way to get pure estradiol is through a compounding pharmacy. At a compounding pharmacy other delivery systems such as sublingual drops and troches are available in any dose you need. The names of all these compounded preparations will be estradiol (sometimes they will be abbreviated as E2).
- I don't recommend estradiol creams or gels that are rubbed on the skin. The absorption is erratic and compliance is low using estradiol this way. It is very easy to forget your doses or to feel too tired to bother rubbing it on correctly!
- Don't use either estriol or estrone in place of estradiol. Neither of these two naturally occurring estrogens is missing in menopause;

─────────

*An exception can be seen in older women who have been in menopause for greater than five years. Some women have burned out their FSH response and will have low levels in menopause.

therefore, they should not be taken as replacement therapy.

• Never use birth control pills as hormone replacement therapy.

• Selective estrogen receptor modulators or S.E.R.M drugs are also not acceptable to be used as estradiol replacement therapy. Don't be fooled by the promises of what these drugs do. These drugs are much more harmful than not taking any hormone replacement therapy.

Dosage and Scheduling: ————————————————————————————————

• In the case of replacing estradiol and progesterone (see progesterone section, too) in a menopausal woman with a uterus, the hormones are replaced to mimic the normal menstrual cycle. If you have a uterus you will be taking estradiol every day and taking progesterone for 11 to 14 days a month. This is known as cycling therapy.

• If you have had a hysterectomy, you may only need to be on estradiol. This depends on whether or not you are still able to make some progesterone and whether or not you feel like something is missing if you are not cycling. Refer to the progesterone section on page 157.

• A good starting dose for a noncompounded estradiol pill is 0.5mg twice a day if you swallow it and 0.5mg cut in half (0.25 mg) if you put it under your tongue and let it dissolve there. I prefer that you try to avoid swallowing estradiol pills because they get filtered through the liver before reaching your blood stream, which is not physiologic.

• A good starting dose for a sublingual (under the tongue) compounded estradiol preparation is 0. 25mg to 0.375mg twice a day.

• I usually only recommend patches be used if you have had your uterus removed (hysterectomy) and the starting dose is 0.025 to 0.05mg changed every 3 and 1/2 days. The reason for this is that anytime the patch falls off, you may experience estradiol withdrawal bleeding. However, don't change if it works for you and feel free to try it if you want to.

Monitoring: ————————————————————————————————

- Monitor how you feel including your sense of well-being and, if you have a uterus, track your monthly withdrawal bleeding. You read that right, you will experience a withdrawal period when your hormones are replaced. This does not mean that you are fertile again!

- The rate of bone loss through urine testing, blood cholesterol levels and the thickness of your uterine lining should be followed by your physician, if applicable.

- If you have a uterus, initially follow your fasting blood levels of estradiol, progesterone and FSH every few months until the hormones are balanced. After that, they should be monitored at least every six months to one year. You must have your blood levels drawn on one of the last three to four days of the progesterone part of the cycle. A general rule of thumb is that your estradiol level should be at the low end of the normal luteal phase range and your FSH level should be approximately half of the starting FSH level (before HRT started). For example, if your FSH started off at 50, you would aim for a level around 25. These recommendations are generalized and may not pertain to you. You may need more or less estradiol to achieve the wanted effects of regular menstrual flow, normalization of cholesterol levels, reversal of bone loss as measured in the urine as well as a feeling of well-being and normalization of sleep patterns. (Refer back to page 159 for progesterone recommendations.)

- You can check your estradiol and FSH levels at anytime if you don't have a uterus and you are not cycling. If you are not cycling, aim for a FSH level at the high normal range of the follicular phase.

- I do not recommend following estradiol levels through saliva samples, as I have not found them to correlate with blood levels from a good lab or with the clinical situation.

If you do not take enough estradiol, you will continue to have the same symptoms you started with and/or you can have fluctuating estradiol levels and become even more symptomatic. If you are taking too much estradiol, you can end up with one or more of the following problems. Note that all of these are identical to the common problems seen when progesterone is too low. Have your levels checked to distinguish between the two.

- Acne
- Arthritic-like pains
- Breast tenderness and/or enlargement
- Decreased memory and/or concentration
- Decreased sex drive
- Depression/irritability
- Dry skin
- Fatigue
- Hair loss
- Headaches
- High blood pressure
- Hot flashes/night sweats
- Irregular or excessive uterine bleeding, especially with increased clots—may also be caused by nonhormonal problems such as fibroids, adenomyosis or polyps
- Mood swings
- PMS
- Vaginal dryness
- Water retention
- Weight gain around the midsection

Testosterone

Who should be tested for testosterone deficiency? Any man over the age of fifty, any man who is on a statin medication (a type of cholesterol lowering drug) or any man with several of the following problems:

Common Symptoms or Problems Associated with Testosterone Deficiency:

- Decreased memory and/or concentration
- Decreased sex drive
- Depression
- Excess weight around the midsection
- High blood sugar levels
- High cholesterol levels
- Loss of bone mass
- Loss of lean body tissue despite adaptive/resistance exercises
- Low energy
- Problem with getting or maintaining erections
- Sleep problems
- Weakness

Or women who have had their ovaries removed, have been in menopause for longer than five years or are taking HRT and despite having normal estradiol and progesterone levels do not feel quite right. Women, it is important to note that the most important hormone for your sex drive is estradiol. Second is progesterone. Balance those hormones first and then replace testosterone if still needed.

The Tests: ————————————————————————————————

Men: Have your free, not total testosterone levels measured as well as a LH level.

Women: Have your free, not total testosterone levels measured but only after your estradiol and progesterone levels are balanced.

Results: ————————————————————————————————

- **Men:** If your free testosterone level is low and your LH level is high you are in male menopause and qualify for testosterone therapy.
- If your free testosterone is low but your LH is low or normal, you have another reason for your low testosterone. You will need to undergo further evaluation. If other reversible causes are not found, you can try testosterone therapy, too.
- **Women:** If your free testosterone levels are below normal you qualify for testosterone therapy as long as you have enough estradiol and progesterone in your body first. If your testosterone levels are low or normal and you still feel awful, you qualify for a trial of low dose testosterone therapy.

The Correct (identical) Hormone: ————————————————

- The bioidentical hormone for testosterone is testosterone. For men this comes in gel and patches found at your local pharmacy. Unfortunately for women lower doses of testosterone are found only at compounding pharmacies.
- Do not use methyltestosterone products or any other synthetic drug testosterone derivative. Some drugs with these are Estratest, Estratest HS, Android capsules, Testred and Virilon. These are not bioidentical testosterone and have many unwanted side effects including abnormal cholesterol levels and increased risk of liver tumors.
- In general I don't recommend testosterone injections. Though they are bioidentical, they tend to create erratic swings in testosterone blood levels causing symptoms such as mood swings and hot flashes for both men and women. However, if you are on testosterone injections and they work for you there is no reason to switch.

Dosage and Scheduling: ————————————————————

- **Men** have higher testosterone levels in the morning and therefore should theoretically take higher amounts of testosterone in the morning. Men need different amounts of testosterone depending on the method of delivery. I will leave this one to your primary care physician. The key is to track the dose you are on with blood levels and adjust accordingly.
- **Women** do not have a significant diurnal variation of this hormone and can take the same small amounts of testosterone in the morning and night. Start with compounded sublingual testosterone at a dosage somehwere between 0.125mg and 2.5mg twice a day. Adjust as needed.

Monitoring: ————————————————————————————

- Watch for side effects of too much testosterone.
- Men, have your free testosterone and LH levels checked in the morning before taking the next dose of testosterone. You want testosterone levels to be at the low end of normal to the mid range at this time of day. You also want your LH levels to be within the normal range.
- Sex hormone binding globulin (SHBG) is another blood test that is used to follow testosterone therapy. If it is too high, you may need more testosterone. If it is too low, you may need less testosterone. This is determined by evaluating your hormone levels of testosterone and LH and the expected effects of the therapy. This requires working with a health care provider well versed in testosterone therapy.
- Women, check your free testosterone and SHBG levels in the morning before your next dose of testosterone. You want your testosterone levels to be at the low end of normal and your SHBG to be within the normal range.

Side Effects of Too Much Testosterone Include:

Men and Women

• Acne
• Hair loss (male pattern baldness)
• Irritability
• Oily skin and hair
• Revved up sex drive
• Weight gain around the midsection
• Worsening versus improvement of cholesterol ratios

Men Only

• Priapism (constant erection)

Women Only

• Abnormal hair growth on your face and/or body
• Deepening of the voice
• Enlargement of the clitoris
• Irregular uterine bleeding
• Too much muscle mass

The Importance of Working with a Health Care Provider Who Specializes in Hormone Systems

I hope that you have come to understand the importance of taking HRT correctly and also realize that taking HRT is a serious endeavor which should only be undertaken with the help of a medical professional well versed in all hormone systems. The goal is not to fill the "tank" back up with the missing hormone but to make sure that the interactions between all hormone systems are recognized, followed and acted on appropriately.

It is critical to have your hormone levels checked before and while on

HRT. The signs and symptoms of hormone problems overlap and it isn't always easy to determine which hormone is out of balance. It is extremely important that you balance out any hormone system that is malfunctioning or you will never have an efficient metabolism.

You have just completed learning about the individual steps of The Schwarzbein Principle Program. Before getting to the specific plans of this program, you will learn what you will go through and what you can expect when you incorporate this Program as a way of life and begin to transition yourself toward health.

PART III

The Schwarzbein Plans

Ten

The Path to Balance

T he Schwarzbein Principle Program is a step-by-step guide to achieving your optimal health, body composition and lifespan. Since the results are dependent on the *current* state of your metabolism, the length of time it takes to affect these changes is different for everyone.

Like any program, the more unhealthy you are to begin with, the more precisely and carefully you will need to follow the program. That is why I have devised two different plans for the Schwarzbein Principle Program.

If you have a damaged metabolism, you will need to begin on the Healing Plan, which has very strict guidelines. After you have healed your metabolism, you will switch to the Maintenance Plan, where you will enjoy a few more liberties once you have reached your ideal body composition.

For those of you with a healthy metabolism, you will begin on the Maintenance Plan. Remember, though, that this plan will only work if you make it a way of life. The good news is that, since you are starting from a relatively healthy place, the results you will see both in your health and your fat weight will occur faster and be more dramatic than among those who begin from an unhealthy starting point.

The Transition

In order to balance your hormones, heal your metabolism and obtain optimum health, you will need to go through a *transition process*. The transition is a journey of re-balancing your hormones and healing if needed. You can only be in your transition if you are improving your nutrition and lifestyle habits through the Schwarzbein Principle Program.

The time it takes to go through the transition is different for everyone. It may take months, or it may take much longer. If you begin with a badly damaged metabolism, it may take years to completely heal. But you *can* heal. It is never too late. You just need to be patient and follow the Healing Plan.

The Four Main Stages of the Transition

1. The Starting Point
2. The Healing Phase
3. The Fat-Burning Phase
4. The Healed State

Let's look at each stage of the process in more detail.

The Starting Point

You either have a healthy metabolism or a damaged metabolism. Take the quiz beginning on page 183 to determine this.

The Healing Phase

Only those who start off with a damaged metabolism will experience a healing phase. In the healing phase your body repairs itself from the damage caused by years of poor nutrition and lifestyle habits. This is a rebuilding time.

It may seem as if you are in suspended animation during this phase because though you are healing, it doesn't always feel or seem that way. As you improve your habits, you are rebuilding your chemicals at a much higher rate than you are using them up, and this doesn't always feel good.

Unfortunately, your body will not start working efficiently the moment you improve your habits. As previously stated, you did not damage your metabolism overnight, and you will not heal it overnight. During the healing phase, you are still hormonally out of balance. As your body begins to correct this imbalance, you may experience any number of disturbing symptoms.

You may feel withdrawal symptoms such as fatigue, irritability and headaches or experience an increase in depression or fluid retention. You may even gain fat weight on a temporary basis. The more damaged your current metabolism is, the longer you will be in the healing phase and the more fat your body is capable of producing and storing. As awful as this may sound, this is your body's only way to heal. So do not be put off by the healing phase—it is a reflection of the damage that came before it, not the program itself.

Unfortunately, even though you begin to improve your habits, the damage has already been done by your previous poor habits. Therefore, you will not instantly reap the rewards of your better habits.

For example, when people stop dieting, they may gain a lot of fat weight and feel tired and listless. They usually tell me they never should have stopped dieting because now they feel lousy and are fat besides.

What they don't realize is that the only way their bodies can heal is by rebuilding, so they will gain fat weight as their bodies heal from years of not eating well. The damage occurred while they were not eating, not after they stopped. The only way to avoid having to heal from dieting is to never diet in the first place.

The Self-Medicating Phase

There is a subpart to the healing phase: the self-medicating phase. If your metabolism is severely damaged, you will probably need to use either toxic chemicals or exercise in order to keep you feeling good enough to continue working on eating and sleeping well. The idea is to do so in a way that keeps you healing and does the least harm.

Because your rebuilding rate must be higher than your using up rate, it does not always feel very good to be in the healing phase of your transition. It is during this time that self-medicating becomes important in keeping you on your path to restoring your metabolism.

In this phase, which occurs simultaneously with the healing phase, you continue to use one or more of the following to make yourself feel good enough to keep up your healing process: stimulants, alcohol, nicotine and/or refined sugars. Overexercising can also be used as a form of self-medication. Self-medicating makes you feel better in the short-term because using up your chemicals always feels better than rebuilding them.

In the self-medicating phase, you are still rebuilding at a faster rate than using up but you narrow the gap between these two processes. Although you prolong your transition, it is sometimes necessary to self-medicate to get through your transition, especially if you begin with a very damaged metabolism. The Healing Plan outlines the best ways to self-medicate if you need to.

Do not make the mistake of thinking you are healing if you have not changed any of your habits! You cannot "be good" part of the time

and revert to your poor habits the rest of the time. If you over self-medicate, you will no longer be in your transition process—you will not be on the plan at all—and you will continue to damage your metabolism.

> As you go through your transition process, remember these points.
>
> • It is never too late to heal, but it does take time.
> • There are no shortcuts so stop looking for them!
> • You must eat well to build well and be well.
> • You must be healthy to lose weight, not lose weight to be healthy.

The Fat-Burning Phase

The fat-burning phase occurs after your body has done all its rebuilding in the healing phase. You begin your fat-burning phase only after your hormones are completely normalized and your metabolism is healed. During this phase you will be rebuilding and using up your functional and structural chemicals at an equal rate. You lose your excess fat weight by using your fat stores as energy to help you regenerate. This is why you must be healthy to lose weight, not lose weight to be healthy.

If you have been following the Healing Plan, this is the stage where you switch to the Maintenance Plan.

The Healed State

The healed state is when all of your hormones are balanced, your metabolism has healed and you have achieved your ideal body composition. You are now through your transition. When you are in this state, you are rebuilding as many chemicals as you are using up, have the body composition you want and have the lowest risk for the

degenerative diseases of aging. Remember, though, that this is a program for life. You must stay on the Schwarzbein Principle Program Maintenance Plan even in the healed state; if you slip back into unhealthy habits, your body will slip back into an unhealthy condition.

Your Current Metabolic State

If you like, you may have your baseline metabolism evaluated through my Web site at *www.schwarzbeinprinciple.com*, but another good way to estimate the state of your metabolism—and therefore the one we'll use here—is to evaluate the current state of your health. Because your weight is not generally a factor in determining the health of your metabolism it is not a criteria. However, excess fat weight around your midsection is a factor, since it is always the result of an unhealthy imbalance in the body.

On the next page is a list of common conditions in our current culture. If you mark any of the choices below, you have a damaged metabolism and you will be following the SPP Healing Plan. If you have none of the conditions below, follow the SPP Maintenance Plan.

Do You Have a Damaged Metabolism?

❑ Addicted to refined sugars, caffeine, nicotine, alcohol or illicit drugs

❑ Allergies, including chronic sinus problems or asthma that require medical treatment

❑ Anxiety disorder or depression requiring medication

❑ Autoimmune disorders such as eczema, endometriosis, lupus, multiple sclerosis, Crohn's disease, ulcerative colitis and rheumatioid arthritis

❑ Candida (systemic)

❑ Chronic degenerative disease of aging such as Alzheimer's disease, Parkinson's, cholesterol abnormalities, heart disease (especially congestive heart failure or heart attack), high blood pressure, osteoarthritis, osteoporosis, plaque in any of your arteries, Type II diabetes, and stroke.

❑ Chronic fatigue syndrome or fibromyalgia

❑ Chronic pain from an unknown source

❑ Excess weight around your midsection associated with cholesterol problems, heart disease, high blood pressure, gout, stroke or Type II diabetes

❑ Excessive fatigue requiring bed rest or stimulants

❑ Heartburn requiring daily medication that is not due to an acute GI infection

❑ Hypoglycemia not related to eating poorly

❑ Insomnia (chronic)

❑ Irritable bowel syndrome

❑ Leaky gut syndrome

❑ Metabolic syndrome (insulin resistance with any of the following: high blood pressure, high uric acid, high triglyceride, low HDL cholesterol levels, obesity, plaque in the heart, neck or brain arteries, or Type II diabetes)

❏ Migraine headaches (chronic)

❏ Premenstrual syndrome lasting most of the month (breast tenderness, water retention *and* emotional changes)

❏ Severe constipation (inability to have *any* bowel movements without laxatives, enemas or stimulants)

❏ Sleep apnea

❏ Stein-Leventhal syndrome (polycystic ovarian syndrome or PCOS)

❏ Ulcer disease (chronic)

Circle the correct statement:

I have a healthy metabolism and will follow the SPP Maintenance Plan.

I have a damaged metabolism and will follow the SPP Healing Plan.

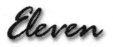

Your Personal Assessment

In general, the SPP steps should be tackled in their stated numerical order. Healthy nutrition is the first step because you will be using food to help you rebuild from past years of breaking down and to help with the other steps of the program. For example, it is important to eat consistently well to help you handle your stresses better, sleep through the night, improve your brain chemistry so you can stop self-medicating with toxic chemicals and supply you with the proper nutrition to sustain an exercise program.

The second step is stress management including sleep because this step helps you slow the using up process, keeps you from needing to self-medicate as much and provides you with the time your body needs to rebuild.

Steps 3 and 4 are also important to help you build efficiently but they are also the steps used as self-medication—using caffeine and stimulating exercises for energy and mood—and therefore should only be fully addressed after you are eating and sleeping well first.

Not everyone will need hormone replacement therapy, which is why it is Step 5. However, Step 5 becomes as important as Steps 1 and 2 if a hormone is missing.

Of course, there are exceptions to all rules—even in my step-by-step program. For some of you, it will be more important to handle your stresses first in order to eat better, and not crave comfort foods, etc. Therefore, Steps 1 and 2 are reversible if you have a serious problem with stress. However, you can make changes that improve your nutrition and stress/sleep habits at the same time. Ideally you will work on eating well and sleeping better simultaneously.

Steps 3 and 4 are also interchangeable, depending on your personal self-medication needs. You can tackle them in either order or together, *but only after Steps 1 and 2 have been addressed.*

If you are having problems mastering Steps 1 and 2 and are making little progress after one month, you may have a hormone problem. Consider Step 5 and get yourself tested.

Don't try to stop toxic chemicals or exercising too much before you have improved your nutrition and stress. If you aren't currently exercising, don't start until you are well nourished and well rested. Making any of these errors will inevitably lead to failure.

Identify Your Personal Challenges

Before you begin to change your nutrition and lifestyle habits, it is time to do a personal assessment. This will not only identify the areas that you will need to work on the most, but it can also alert you to major problems that will necessitate switching the order of some steps. Remember, it is best to follow the steps in order, so only make changes if you feel there is a serious issue you need to address.

Check all of the following that apply to you. Be honest and objective. If you cannot answer no to a particular question, or you don't understand it, assume you need to address that step as part of your healing process and check it off.

Step 1: Nutrition

Consider this step a high priority if you check off the first point. Checking all three points means you are doing extremely poorly with nutrition.

❑   I do not eat correctly. (Eating correctly means eating a balanced diet of three meals and at least one snack consisting of quality proteins, real carbohydrates, healthy fats and nonstarchy vegetables.

❑   I drink too many glasses of milk or fruit juices. (If you have a healthy metabolism, it is acceptable to drink one glass of milk or fresh fruit juice on a daily basis. If you have a damaged metabolism, you should not be having any.)

❑   I do not drink at least the equivalent of six, eight-ounce glasses of water a day (including herbal teas and sparkling waters).

Step 2: Stress Management

If you did not check the first blank in nutrition and any of the first four points below are checked, you should consider working on your stress management first.

❑   I have stress that interferes with my health.

❑   I do not handle stresses well. Emotionally, this means that I get easily upset over small issues. Physically, it means that my stresses are interfering with my vital signs, my appetite or my sleep pattern.

❑   I am too busy or work too many hours to take care of all my personal needs, including eating well, sleeping and exercising consistently.

❑   I do not get at least eight hours of uninterrupted sleep a night.

❑   I do not have enough downtime in my day.

❑   I do not incorporate stress management techniques into my life.

❑   I don't feel like I am ever stressed. (This is a trick question. If you checked this box, you are either in denial, very lucky or dead. Please rethink all of your answers above. If you still don't believe you are stressed, you won't have to work on stress management.)

Step 3: Avoiding Toxic Chemicals

If you have a healthy metabolism, small amounts of caffeine, alcohol and refined sugars throughout the week will not break this program. If you have a damaged metabolism, you need to taper off most of these chemicals at your own pace until your metabolism has improved. This step only becomes a priority after the first two steps are addressed. An exception is if you are addicted to an illegal drug or alcohol.

❑   I am addicted to illegal drugs, painkillers or alcohol—please stop reading this book now and look into a rehab program.

❑   I use tobacco products.

❑   I drink more than one beer or half a glass of wine three times a week.

❑   I routinely take prescription medications. (Do not count hormones such as thyroid, insulin or estradiol.)

❑   I routinely take over-the-counter medications. (This includes but is not limited to allergy, heartburn, arthritis and headache medications.)

❑   I use artificial sugars.

❑   I eat/drink refined sugars in a typical day (such as desserts, candy and sodas).

❑   I ingest additives, chemical preservatives and other fake chemicals.

❑   I drink more than two caffeinated cups of coffee or tea in one day.

Step 4: Smart Exercise

A smart exercise program consists of a combination of calming/stretching, and adaptive/resistance plus or minus stimulating/cardiovascular exercises. If you have a damaged metabolism, you should not be doing any stimulating exercises. If you are over-exercising, you need to tackle Step 4 before Step 3. An exception is if you are using exercise as a form of self-medication.

❏ I exercise strenuously on a daily basis.

❏ I get either hyped up or tired from exercise, not energized.

❏ I am not eating and sleeping well before I exercise. (Eating well means not skipping meals, eating real foods, and balancing proteins and carbohydrates. Sleeping well means getting at least eight hours of uninterrupted sleep the night before.)

❏ I do stimulating/cardiovascular exercises more than three times a week.

❏ I do not do any adaptive/resistance training.

❏ I do not have a consistent exercise routine that includes three to five sessions a week.

Step 5: Hormone Replacement Therapy

Since all hormone systems are interconnected, one missing hormone can keep you from achieving optimum health. If a hormone is low or missing and your body will never be able to make it again, for example the loss of estradiol (the human estrogen made by the ovaries) in menopause, you need to take that hormone to be in full balance. If you check any of the blanks below, Step 5 becomes an integral part of your program as it can be as important as all the other steps combined. You need to work on HRT at the same time you are working on eating and sleeping well.

❏ I have a glandular hormone problem and do not take HRT (this includes menopause).

❏ I have a glandular hormone problem and take hormone replacement therapy (insulin, thyroid, DHEA, sex hormones, cortisol, Human Growth Hormone, etc.).

❏ I take HRT but not the way described in Chapter 9. I am not taking a bioidentical form of HRT in such a way as to mimic the normal production and secretion of the hormone deficiency I am being treated for.

❏ I do not know whether I have a hormone problem that requires hormone replacement therapy.

NOTE: *Besides hormone replacement therapy for hormone deficiencies, you will also need to address hormone excesses caused by glandular problems before you can be in balance. This is too complicated an issue for this book, so I will leave it up to your primary physician to either treat the issue or refer you to someone who can.*

This checklist of your personal challenges can help you prioritize the five steps of your Schwarzbein Principle Program. Review your check marks for each section to determine if you need to address any step in a special order. Remember that only Steps 1 or 2 are interchangeable; that Steps 3 and 4 are interchangeable only after completing Steps 1 and 2; and that Step 5 is as important as Steps 1 and 2 if you need to take HRT. Fill in the following blanks with the order of how you will personally follow the five-step program.

1. Step _____
2. Step_____
3. Step_____
4. Step_____
5. Step_____

I hope that the above exercise opened your eyes to the lifestyle changes you need to make to become healthy, energetic and ideally suited to your body. Now it is time to give you the prescription—the Schwarzbein Principle Program Plans—that will help make this happen.

Twelve

The Healing Plan

The Schwarzbein Principle Program (SPP) Healing Plan has been specifically designed to help you repair your metabolism by making positive changes to your nutrition and lifestyle habits. How long this will take is different for everyone. The worse your metabolism, the longer it will take to heal. The good news is that if you are willing to make the necessary changes, you will be much healthier in one year's time than you are right now.

You will go through a transition period that is unavoidable, necessary and at times somewhat uncomfortable. Healing is a time of rebuilding. If you stick with it and get through the healing phase, the reward is a healthier life than you ever thought possible.

Please make sure you are following the right plan for you. The Healing Plan should only be followed by those of you who need to heal their metabolism. Following the SPP Healing Plan when you don't have to heal can cause damage to your metabolism. Needing to lose weight does not necessarily equate with needing to heal. If you only have to lose fat weight, not heal your metabolism, follow the Maintenance Plan.

Remember to follow these steps in the order you determined in

your personal assessment. If you skip ahead, you not only risk relapse but you will not get the full benefits of the Program.

Step 1: Healthy Nutrition, including taking supplements if needed

Basic Requirement:

- Eat five "squares" of quality protein (low in long chain saturated fats), real carbohydrates, the recommended amounts of healthy fats and nonstarchy vegetables a day; eat three meals and two snacks. If you find that this is too much food at a sitting, it is acceptable to divide the total food for the day into smaller portions and eat six or more times a day.
- Do *not* skip meals or count calories. This is not a low-calorie diet.
- Follow the prescribed eating requirements for each food group.
- Use the 12 supplements listed on a daily basis (recommended, not required).

The SPP Healing Plan *requires* you to eat smaller portions more frequently, but it is not a low-calorie diet. If you don't eat enough food you won't have the necessary material needed to rebuild and repair. If you eat too much food at a given moment, you will overbuild. On this plan, you will be eating plenty of food, just spreading it out more evenly.

Do not skip meals or snacks. I understand that making the time to eat more frequently can be hard to do, but this is one of the most important things you will be doing for yourself on a daily basis.

Because you have a damaged metabolism, your appetite is not always the best way to determine how much you should be eating. You must follow the recommended guidelines for your total protein and carbohydrate intake. This will ensure that you have the minimum food requirements needed to help you rebuild and repair. If you gain a lot of fat weight when you begin eating better, you have a very

damaged metabolism. Do not go back to your bad habits and cut back on portion sizes, skip meals or go on a popular diet to lose this weight. You will destroy your metabolism further in the long run if you do.

You have to eat well to heal your metabolism. Once you have healed your metabolism, you will never have to diet again—your body will burn fat efficiently without your needing to lower your caloric intake.

For at least one to three months, you will be following a gluten free diet. Gluten, a protein found in most grains (see list Appendix B, page 260) causes an allergic reaction in at least 1 out of every 30 Americans (ranging from mild to full-blown celiac disease) that, among many problems, destroys your metabolism. Since you have to heal your metabolism, you want to follow a no-gluten plan until you can sort out whether or not you have a true problem with gluten. If you are allergic to gluten and eat it, you will not be able to lose fat weight or feel better. Even worse, you will not be able to heal your metabolism.

You will need to stay off of gluten for the rest of your life if you find out you have a gluten intolerance. If you are from English, Irish, Welsh, Scottish, Scandinavian or Eastern European descent, you are most likely to end up with a permanent gluten intolerance.

General Nutrition Guidelines:

If you do not eat well, your metabolism will never heal. The purpose of eating is to rebuild. You cannot rebuild your body chemicals if you skip meals, do not eat enough food, do not eat the right balance of foods, eat damaged or junk food or drink instead of eat your meals.

Refer to the food lists in Chapter 5: Nutrition for acceptable foods in each category.

Protein Requirements:
Men:
- 13 to 23 ounces per day:
  3 to 5 ounces (21 to 35 grams) with meals; 2 to 4 ounces (14 to 28 grams) with snacks.

Women:
- 8 to 18 ounces per day:
  2 to 4 ounces (14 to 28 grams) with meals; 1 to 3 ounces (7 to
  21 grams) with snacks

In general, the taller you are, the more you weigh and the more active you are, the higher your protein needs. It is also acceptable to simply divide the total ounces evenly between the five meal times.

Protein Requirement Calculations

If you wish, you can calculate protein requirements for your specific sex, body type and activity level by following the instructions provided in Appendix A on page 254.

Quality Protein Portions

You can approximate your protein portion requirement by sight. One ounce of protein is approximately ¼ the size of your palm and as thick as a deck of a cards. The food equivalent is:

1 ounce lean ground sirloin, lean cuts of lamb and pork, chicken, turkey, and fish

1 egg

1 ounce canned tuna (⅙ of can)

¼ cup organic lowfat cottage cheese

1 ounce organic skim milk mozzarella, feta or goat cheese

⅜ cup tofu

¼ cup tempeh

Nuts: ⅛ cup edamame, 1 ounce almonds, 1½ ounce other nuts

Use these quantities to determine the amount you should eat for each protein portion. For instance, if you want to eat three ounces of protein, simply multiply the portions above by three.

Carbohydrate Requirements:

Eat gluten-free carbohydrates for at least the first one to three months of the Healing Plan in the quantities described:

- One hundred and twenty-five grams of carbohydrates per day; 25 grams per sitting
- If you have Type II diabetes or the metabolic syndrome: 100 grams of carbohydrates a day; 20 per sitting.
- If you are Extremely Active (see Appendix A page 256): 175 grams of carbohydrates per day; 35 per sitting until you taper down to Very Active and then eat 150 grams of carbohydrates per day; 30 per sitting.
- If you are Very Active *and* have Type II diabetes or the metabolic syndrome (you should not be Extremely Active if you have one of these conditions): 125 grams of carbohydrates per day; 25 grams per sitting.
- One serving of a low glycemic index fruit a day, if desired, but only as part of a snack, not a meal.

If you are appalled at the "high" amount of carbohydrates per meal, you have succumbed to the false promises of one of the popular diets promoting too few carbohydrates. If you don't eat enough carbohydrates, you send signals to your body that it is in the middle of a famine causing your body to "eat" its own lean muscle tissue for energy. Decreasing your carbohydrate intake too low causes "starvation" weight loss at first, but increases the probability that you will gain fat weight in the long term.

Fat Requirements:
- Plenty of monounsaturated and short chain saturated fats.
- Small amounts of healthy polyunsaturated fats.
- Three grams or less per meal of foods that contain long chain saturated fats.
- Avoid all damaged fats (transfatty acids, rancid fats, partially hydrogenated oils and fully hydrogenated fats).

You will be severely limiting but not eliminating your saturated fat intake on the basic Healing Plan diet. However, if you have high blood sugars, high triglyceride levels or high blood pressure disease, you may want to restrict your saturated fats even further. Only do this if you are not responding to the basic meal plans and guidelines. If the basic plan is not working, follow the low saturated fat meal plans.

Nonstarchy Vegetable Requirements:

- Minimum of 5 cups a day; one cup serving at meals and ½ cup serving at snacks.

Don't be shy about nonstarchy vegetables. The more you eat the better. Do not count these as carbohydrates. A nonstarchy vegetable is any portion of a half cup that contains five grams or less of carbohydrate. Make sure that you are eating a variety of nonstarchy vegetables and rotate them to avoid developing food allergies and to reap the benefits from the different plant chemicals.

Supplement Requirements:

It is highly recommended *but not required* that you take all of the following supplements to help heal your metabolism. They also help with problems such as carbohydrate cravings, low mood and low energy as well as help jump-start fat weight loss.

- A good twice-a-day multivitamin and mineral.
- High quality omega fish oils.
- Stress B complex.
- Calcium and magnesium at bedtime.
- Carnitine.
- Chromium (not a picolinate form).
- Coenzyme Q-10.
- Glutamine.
- Lipoic acid.
- Taurine.
- Vitamin C.
- Vitamin E as mixed tocopherols.

These 12 supplements are what I recommend for basic healing. Unfortunately, they are not always enough if you have a severely damaged metabolism to target all your specific needs. Please refer to the supplement information in Chapter 5: Nutrition if you feel you could benefit from additional supplements.

Six Helpful Hints to Changing Food Habits

1. Do not invite the enemy to the table

- If you are served a breadbasket, ask the waitperson to remove it from the table.
- Don't order foods you should not be eating such as pizza and pasta dishes.
- Don't keep bad food choices stocked at home. In fact this is a great time to go through your cupboards and clean out all the "non-foods" that are not on this plan
- Ask your friends and family to be courteous and not flaunt your favorite junk food in your face or eat it when you are around.

2. The 3-bite rule for special occasions

- If you feel that you must have something on a special occasion that is not on your plan follow the 3-bite rule and only have three small bites. This is not the same as when you give in to an out-of-control craving.

3. Speak up when dining at someone's home

- Start by asking them what they are making so you know whether or not you will be able to eat it. Then, depending on your level of comfort, ask them to make you something different if it doesn't fit your plan or bring your own food. Once my friends and family knew what I expected to be fed, they would plan a healthy meal around the things that I could eat. This way all the other guests got a healthier meal, too!

Six Helpful Hints to Changing Food Habits (cont'd)

4. **Don't feel guilty if you are not perfect**
   * The changes you are making take time. This is a process. I guarantee you will not be able to be perfect all the time. But if you concentrate on not skipping meals and eating balanced meals, I give you my word that eating this way will get easier and easier until you no longer have to think about it.
5. **Think ahead when traveling or at work**
   * It is guaranteed that you will not get served real food when you travel. Take mixed nuts with or without raisins for snacks and bring food from home to eat on the plane.
   * Buy yourself a cooler and keep staple foods in it for when you are traveling in the car.
   * At work, stock the company refrigerator with healthy foods and bring your lunch with you.
6. **Journal your food, mood and exercise intake.** It has been shown that keeping a food and lifestyle journal helps keep you accountable and helps you make changes to your habits faster and permanently. You can download food, mood and exercise diary sheets off my website at *http://www.schwarzbeinprinciple.com/ pgs/dr_schw/institute1.html* or create your own.

Meal Plans

Create your own meal plans by following these four recommendations or follow the predesigned meal plans starting on page 202:

1. Choose a quality protein, one that is also low in long chain saturated fat.
2. Include real carbohydrates.
3. Eat a variety of nonstarchy vegetables throughout the day, as much as you like.
4.) Add healthy fats in moderate amounts.

In general it should take approximately two to six weeks to make the necessary changes to your meal plans including drinking enough water. Remember that this is your personal transition process and you should make the necessary changes to your health as quickly or as slowly as necessary to make this a permanent lifestyle modification.

If you find you are having a difficult time making the necessary changes, I highly recommend that you take the suggested supplements. If that doesn't help, work with a food coach or dietitian for accountability and suggestions. Or consider that stress or hormone problems may be keeping you from making these changes.

Start by following the gluten–free meal and snack plans for at least one month if not more. If you don't feel that you have a gluten problem, switch to the lower saturated fat plans. Mix and match the meals and snacks but try to rotate your foods and not eat the same thing day in and day out. You will find the 30 gram carbohydrate selections in the Maintenance Plan, if needed.

20 gram Gluten Free Sample Menu Plan

Each meal contains approximately 20 grams of carbohydrates

MEALS	MONDAY	TUESDAY	WEDNESDAY	THURSDAY	FRIDAY	SATURDAY	SUNDAY
Breakfast	Burrito: Eggs, muenster cheese, avocado slices, chopped tomato wrapped in a medium corn tortilla	3/4 cup cream of rice w/cinnamon and crushed walnuts String cheese *Carrot sticks	Scoop of eggless egg salad (made from tofu) on Nut Thins (15 crackers) *Sliced tomatoes	Scrambled eggs Fresh salsa 1/4 cup black beans 1 small corn tortilla	Cottage cheese 1 slice rice bread toast w/organic sugar-free almond butter *raw veggies	Hard boiled egg(s) 1 cup hot amaranth cereal Celery dipped in natural peanut butter	Vegetable scramble: Eggs, broccoli, onions, spinach, and feta cheese 2/3 cup roasted potatoes
Lunch	1 small baked potato stuffed w/1/2 cup cottage cheese and steamed broccoli	Mexican salad: Lettuce, seasoned ground sirloin, 1/2 cup kidney beans, fresh salsa, and guacamole	1 cup plain whole milk yogurt 1 cup air popped popcorn + mixed nuts raw veggies	Scoop of tuna salad (made with chopped onions, celery, and pure pressed oil mayo) 11 Edward & Son brown rice snaps	Grilled salmon Cold bean salad: black beans, kidney beans, corn, tomato, cilantro, garlic, and olive oil tossed together 1/2 cup portion	Chinese chicken salad: mixed greens, shredded cabbage, grilled chicken, and almond slivers Oriental dressing (no added sugar) 1 small jicama, chopped	Turkey sandwich: 1 slice rice bread, nitrate free turkey, lettuce, tomato, onions, pure pressed oil mayonnaise
Dinner	Grilled lamb chops 1/2 c brown rice Grilled zucchini Mixed greens salad w/vinaigrette	Grilled salmon 2/3 c red potatoes Sautéed spinach Chopped cucumber, carrots and tomatoes w/vinaigrette	Stir-fried pork and vegetables served over 1/2 cup buckwheat Add salad if desired	Baked halibut 1 small sweet potato w/a dab of butter Mixed green salad w/vinaigrette	Grilled chicken 1 large artichoke, steamed Broccoli and cauliflower mix Add salad if desired	Tuna Melt: Tuna salad made with pure pressed canola, lettuce, thick slice of tomato, and melted mozzarella on 1 slice rice bread Mixed green salad w/vinaigrette	Steak smothered with sautéed onions, mushrooms, and peppers Small baked potato w/a dab of butter Small Caesar salad, Newman's Caesar dressing, no croutons

1. When bread is indicated, use: Rice Bread; Crackers: Edward & Son (brown rice snaps), Nut Thins, Black Sesame Seed Rice Crackers (Whole Foods); Tortillas: Corn; Dressings: Drew's, Spectrum, Newman's Own Oil & Vinegar and Caesar, Annie's Italian
2. If raw vegetables are indicated, use carrots, celery, onions, cucumber, broccoli, cauliflower, peppers.
3. Mixed greens could include: variety of lettuce, spinach, onions, tomatoes, grated carrots, cucumber, celery, peppers.
4. *If you are a diabetic, raw carrots and tomatoes may cause blood sugar to increase.
5. When butter is indicated, use organic, raw unsweetened, unsalted butter.

25 gram Gluten Free Sample Menu Plan

Each meal contains approximately 25 grams of carbohydrates

MEALS	MONDAY	TUESDAY	WEDNESDAY	THURSDAY	FRIDAY	SATURDAY	SUNDAY
Breakfast	Burrito: Eggs, muenster cheese, avocado slices, chopped tomato wrapped in a large corn tortilla	1cup cream of rice w/ cinnamon and crushed walnuts String cheese *Carrot sticks	Scoop of eggless egg salad (made from tofu) on Nut Thins (18 crackers) *Sliced tomatoes	Scrambled eggs Fresh salsa 1/3 cup black beans 1 small corn tortilla	Cottage cheese 1 slice rice bread toast w/organic sugar-free almond butter *raw veggies	Hard boiled egg(s) 1 1/4 cup hot amaranth cereal Celery dipped in natural peanut butter	Vegetable scramble Eggs, broccoli, onions, spinach, and feta cheese 3/4 cup roasted potatoes
Lunch	1 small baked potato stuffed w/1/2 cup cottage cheese and steamed broccoli	Mexican salad: Lettuce, seasoned ground sirloin, 1/3 cup kidney beans, 1/3 cup corn, fresh salsa, and guacamole	1 cup plain whole milk yogurt 2 cups air popped popcorn + mixed nuts raw veggies	Scoop of tuna salad (made with chopped onions, celery, and pure pressed oil mayo) 13 Edward & Son brown rice snaps	Grilled salmon Cold bean salad: black beans, kidney beans, corn, tomato, cilantro, garlic, and olive oil tossed together: 2/3 cup portion	Chinese chicken salad: mixed greens, shredded cabbage, grilled chicken, and almond slivers Oriental dressing (no sugar added) 1 small jicama, chopped	Turkey sandwich: 1 slice rice bread, nitrate free turkey, lettuce, tomato, onions, pure pressed oil mayonnaise
Dinner	Grilled lamb chops 3/4 cup brown rice Grilled zucchini Mixed greens salad w/vinaigrette	Grilled salmon 1/2 cup red potatoes 1/3 cup corn Sautéed spinach Chopped cucumber, carrots and tomatoes w/ vinaigrette	Stir-fried pork and vegetables served over 1/2 cup buckwheat Add salad if desired	Baked halibut 1 small sweet potato w/ a dab of butter Mixed green salad w/vinaigrette	Grilled chicken 1 large artichoke, steamed Broccoli and cauliflower mix Add salad if desired	Tuna Melt: Tuna salad made with pure pressed canola, lettuce, thick slice of tomato, and melted mozzarella on 1 slice rice bread Mixed green salad w/vinaigrette	Steak smothered with sautéed onions, mushrooms, and peppers Small baked potato w/a dab of butter Small Caesar salad, Newman's Caesar dressing, no croutons

1. When bread is indicated, use: Rice Bread; Crackers: Edward & Son (brown rice snaps), Nut Thins, Black Sesame Seed Rice Crackers (Whole Foods); Tortillas: Corn; Dressings: Drew's, Spectrum, Newman's Own Oil & Vinegar and Caesar, Annie's Italian

2. If raw vegetables are indicated, use carrots, celery, onions, cucumber, broccoli, cauliflower, peppers.

3. Mixed greens could include: variety of lettuce, spinach, onions, tomatoes, grated carrots, cucumber, celery, peppers.

4. *If you are a diabetic, raw carrots and tomatoes may cause blood sugar to increase.

5. When butter is indicated, use organic, raw unsweetened, unsalted butter.

Snack Ideas
Gluten-Free
20 grams Carbohydrates

- 1¼ cups whole strawberries and ricotta cheese
- 1 slice of gluten free bread (20g) and organic sugar-free peanut butter
- 4 Corn Thins with egg salad, tuna salad, or chicken salad
- ½ medium baked potato with mozzarella cheese and fresh salsa
- 3 cups air popped popcorn and mixed nuts
- 1 cup raspberries and cottage cheese
- 1 slice rice, buckwheat, or millet bread (20g) with avocado, and chicken salad
- 1 cup organic, plain, whole milk yogurt, ½ cup strawberries, and crushed walnuts
- 1 slice of gluten free bread (20 g), tomatoes, feta cheese, and carrot sticks
- 15 Nut Thin crackers with almond butter
- 1 slice of rice bread (20g), nitrate free turkey, lettuce, tomato, and mayonnaise (pure pressed oils)
- ½ medium sweet potato and nitrate free chicken sausage
- 10 Edward & Son brown rice snaps, cucumber, and goat cheese
- 2 small corn tortillas (20g), melted mozzarella cheese, avocado, and fresh salsa
- ¾ cup grapefruit and hard boiled egg(s)
- ½ cup hummus with raw vegetables and cashews
- 15 Nut Thin crackers, mozzarella cheese, and spicy mustard
- ¾ cup blueberries and almonds
- 1 cup edemame beans (shelled)

If following the lower saturated fat guidelines: Substitute part-skim mozzarella, low-fat ricotta, low-fat cottage cheese, or reduced fat plain yogurt for any dairy product listed. Eat limited amounts of sausage. Eat limited amounts of sausage.

To round out your snacks, add some non-starchy vegetables such as celery, carrots, tomatoes, cucumbers, peppers, broccoli, snap peas, and cauliflower.

Snack Ideas
Gluten-Free
25 grams Carbohydrates

* 1½ cups whole strawberries and ricotta cheese
* 2 slices of gluten free bread (25g) and organic sugar-free peanut butter
* 5 Corn Thins with egg salad, tuna salad, or chicken salad
* 1 small baked potato with mozzarella cheese and fresh salsa
* 4 cups air popped popcorn and mixed nuts
* 1½ cup raspberries and sunflower seeds
* 1 slice rice, buckwheat, or millet bread (25g) with avocado, and chicken salad
* 1 cup organic, plain, whole milk yogurt, ½ cup blueberries, and crushed walnuts
* 2 slices of gluten free bread (25g), tomatoes, feta cheese, and carrot sticks
* 18 Nut Thin crackers with almond butter
* 1 slice rice bread (25g), nitrate free turkey, lettuce, tomato, and mayonnaise (pure pressed oils)
* 1 small sweet potato and nitrate free chicken sausage
* 13 Edward & Son brown rice snaps, cucumber, and goat cheese
* 2 small corn tortillas (25g), melted mozzarella cheese, avocado, and fresh salsa
* 1 small grapefruit and hard boiled egg(s)
* ½ cup hummus, 5 Nut Thin crackers, raw vegetables, and cashews
* 16 Nut Thin crackers, mozzarella cheese, and spicy mustard
* ¾ cup blueberries and cottage cheese
* 1¼ cup edemame beans (shelled)

If following the lower saturated fat guidelines: Substitute part-skim mozzarella, low-fat ricotta, low-fat cottage cheese, or reduced fat plain yogurt for any dairy product listed. Eat limited amounts of sausage.

To round out your snacks, add some non-starchy vegetables such as celery, carrots, tomatoes, cucumbers, peppers, broccoli, snap peas, and cauliflower.

20 gram Low Saturated Fat Sample Menu Plan

Each meal contains approximately 20 grams of carbohydrates per meal

MEALS	MONDAY	TUESDAY	WEDNESDAY	THURSDAY	FRIDAY	SATURDAY	SUNDAY
Breakfast	Eggs with onions and peppers 1/2 cup black beans Fresh salsa	1 cup oatmeal w/cinnamon, and crushed walnuts Hard boiled egg(s)	Nitrate-free turkey 10 Edward & Son rice snaps w/organic sugar free peanut butter *carrot sticks	Greek omelet w/ spinach, tomatoes, and a few feta crumbles 3/4 cup roasted potatoes	Low fat cottage cheese 1/2 medium jicama, chopped handful of raw mixed nuts *raw veggies	Breakfast burrito: Eggs, tomatoes, and avocado wrapped in a medium/large corn tortilla	Eggs over easy 1 1/2 slice Ezekial toast Celery and organic sugar-free peanut butter
Lunch	Grilled salmon on a bed on spinach, cherry tomatoes, and avocado w/vinaigrette 1/2 cup couscous	1/2 Turkey sandwich: nitrate free turkey, 1 slice ezekial bread, pure pressed oil mayonnaise Chicken (without noodles)	Grilled skinless chicken on mixed greens with 1/2 cup chick peas, green onions, and roasted red peppers w/vinaigrette	Fish taco: 1 medium/large corn tortilla, fish of choice, shredded cabbage, chopped tomatoes, avocado, cilantro, and squeezed lemon	Southwest Salad: Ground seasoned turkey breast, mixed greens, tomatoes, 1/3 cup corn, 1/4 cup black beans, fresh salsa, and guacamole	Tuna melt: Tuna mixed w/ pure pressed oil mayo and sunflower seeds, thick tomato slice, and melted skim-milk mozzarella on 1 slice Vogel bread *raw veggies	Grilled chicken, salmon, or shrimp Caesar salad, no croutons, Newman's Caesar dressing 5 Ak mak crackers
Dinner	Baked skinless chicken breast Asparagus spears 2/3 cup mashed red potatoes Mixed green salad w/vinaigrette	Grilled pork chop w/ sautéed onions 1/2 large sweet potato w/dab of butter Caesar salad, no croutons, Newman's Caesar dressing	Baked red snapper Sautéed mushroom caps in garlic and olive oil 1 cup acorn squash Add salad if desired	Chicken stir fry w/ snap peas, broccoli, bean sprouts, and peppers over 1/2 cup brown rice Hearts of romaine w/Italian (no sugar added)	Grilled shrimp 1 small ear of corn Mixed greens w/tomatoes, cucumbers, olives, sunflower seeds, and vinaigrette	Grilled skinless chicken breast Veggie kabobs w/mushrooms, peppers, and onions 1/2 large baked potato w/ dab of butter Add salad if desired	Sautéed seasoned tofu w/ spinach, garlic, and olive oil 1/2 cup couscous *Chopped cucumber, carrot, and tomato w/vinaigrette

1. When bread is indicated, use: Ezekial, Vogel or Alvarado; Crackers: AkMak, Lavosh, Wasa, Edward & Son (brown rice snaps), 365 Woven Wheats, Nut Pitas: Cedarlane; Tortillas: Corn, Alvarado Street; Dressings: Drew's, Spectrum, Newman's Own Oil & Vinegar and Caesar, Annie's Italian
2. If raw vegetables are indicated, use: carrots, celery, onions, cucumber, broccoli, cauliflower, peppers.
3. Mixed greens could include: variety of lettuce, spinach, onions, tomatoes, grated carrots, cucumber, celery, peppers.
4. *If you are a diabetic, raw carrots and tomatoes may cause blood sugar to increase.
5. When butter is indicated, use organic, unsweetened, unsalted butter.

25 gram Lower Saturated Fat Sample Menu Plan

Each meal contains approximately 25 grams of carbohydrates

MEALS	MONDAY	TUESDAY	WEDNESDAY	THURSDAY	FRIDAY	SATURDAY	SUNDAY
Breakfast	Scoop of eggless egg salad (made w/ tofu) on 7 Ak Mak crackers Sliced tomatoes	Breakfast Burrito: eggs, avocado slices, chopped tomato wrapped in a large corn tortilla	1 1/2 Slices Ezeckial toast w/organic, sugar-free almond butter Skinless chicken breast *carrot sticks	Scrambled eggs Fresh salsa 1/3 cup black beans 1 small corn tortilla	Low fat cottage cheese 18 Nut Thin crackers *raw veggies	Nitrate-free turkey slices 1 1/4 cup oatmeal Celery w/organic, sugar-free peanut butter	Egg Scramble: eggs, spinach, and part-skim mozzarella 3/4c roasted potatoes
Lunch	Fish, shrimp, or chicken tacos: 2 small corn tortillas, diced cabbage, tomato, and avocado served with fresh salsa and squeezed lemon	Turkey burger served w/ lettuce, tomato, sprouts, dijon and pure pressed oil mayo on 2 slices low carb whole grain bread	Mexican Salad: lettuce, seasoned ground turkey breast, 1/3 cup black beans, 1/3 cup corn, fresh salsa, and guacamole	1 medium whole grain pita stuffed w/ sprouts and tuna salad (made with onions, celery, sunflower seeds, and pure pressed oil mayonnaise)	Grilled shrimp, salmon, or chicken Caesar salad, no croutons, Newman's Caesar dressing 3 Wasa hearty rye crisp bread	Chinese Chix Salad: mixed greens, shredded cabbage, grilled chicken, almond slivers, Oriental dressing (without added sugar)	Turkey Sandwich: 2 slices low carb whole grain bread, nitrate free turkey, lettuce, tomato, onions, pure pressed oil mayonnaise
Dinner	Chicken Pita: skinless chicken breast, lettuce, tomato, onion, and pesto basil mayo (made w/ pure pressed oil) in a whole grain pita Add salad if desired	Stir-fried pork and vegetables served on 1/2 cup brown rice Small Caesar salad, no croutons, Newman's Caesar dressing	Grilled sea bass Sauteed spinach, garlic, and olive oil 1 1/4 cup butternut squash Chopped cucumber, carrots and tomatoes w/ vinaigrette	Baked halibut 1 small sweet potato w/ dab of butter Broccoli and cauliflower mix Add salad if desired	Grilled skinless chicken breast 1 large artichoke, steamed dipped in pure pressed oil mayonnaise Mixed green salad w/ Italian dressing	Mushroom barley soup 1/2 tuna sandwich: 1 slice whole grain bread, tuna salad, lettuce, and tomato Add salad if desired	Grilled skinless chicken smothered w/sautéed onions, mushrooms, and peppers Small baked potato w/dab of butter Grilled zucchini Add salad if desired

1. When bread is indicated, use: Ezekial, Vogel or Alvarado; Crackers: AkMak, Lavosh, Wasa, Edward & Son (brown rice snaps), 365 Woven Wheats, Nut Pitas: Cedarlane; Tortillas: Corn, Alvarado Street; Dressings: Drew's, Spectrum, Newman's Own Oil & Vinegar and Caesar, Annie's Italian
2. If raw vegetables are indicated, use: carrots, celery, onions, cucumber, broccoli, cauliflower, peppers.
3. Mixed greens could include: variety of lettuce, spinach, onions, tomatoes, grated carrots, cucumber, celery, peppers.
4. *If you are a diabetic, raw carrots and tomatoes may cause blood sugar to increase.
5. When butter is indicated, use organic, unsweetened, unsalted butter.

Snack Ideas
Low Glycemic Fruits and Lower Saturated Fat
15 grams Carbohydrates

- 1¼ cups strawberries and part-skim milk mozzarella cheese
- 1 nitrate free chicken sausage on a whole grain bread
- ½ grapefruit and walnuts
- ½ medium baked potato and low-fat cottage cheese
- 1 small corn tortilla, nitrate free turkey, shredded lettuce, and mayonnaise
- ½ medium raw jicama and organic sugar-free peanut butter
- 1 small whole wheat tortilla, tomatoes, and feta cheese
- 2½ cups air popped popcorn and mixed nuts
- 3 Finn crisp and egg salad
- 1 cup raspberries and low-fat cottage cheese
- 1 slice whole wheat bread and chicken salad
- 4-6 whole grain crackers, cucumber and goat cheese
- ½ cup blueberries and pecans
- ½ cup hummus, raw carrots/celery, almonds
- ¾ cup edemame beans (unshelled)
- ½ slice of Ezeckial bread with turkey (nitrate free), ham (nitrate free) or tuna salad

To round out your snacks, add some non-starchy vegetables such as celery, carrots, tomatoes, cucumbers, peppers, broccoli, snap peas, and cauliflower.

Snack Ideas
Lower Saturated Fat
20 grams Carbohydrates

- 1½ cups strawberries and skim milk mozzarella cheese
- *1 medium apple and organic, sugar-free peanut butter
- 4 Finn crisps with egg salad, tuna salad, or chicken salad
- *Goat cheese spread on 2 medium apricots
- 3 cups air popped popcorn and mixed nuts
- *⅔ cup unsweetened applesauce and low-fat cottage cheese
- 5 Ak Mak crackers, skim milk mozzarella cheese, and spicy mustard
- *1 medium pear and almonds
- 1 cup organic, plain, reduced-fat yogurt, ½ cup strawberries, and crushed walnuts
- 1 small corn tortilla, tomatoes, feta cheese, and carrot sticks
- *1 cup fresh pineapple and low-fat ricotta cheese
- 1 slice vogel bread with avocado and chicken salad
- ½ medium baked potato with a scoop of low-fat cottage cheese
- 16 Nut Thin crackers, cucumber and goat cheese
- *1 medium orange and pecans
- ½ cup hummus with raw vegetables and almonds
- 1 cup edamame beans (shelled)

———————
*If you have an insulin resistant condition substitute these fruits, ½ cup blueberries, 1 cup other berries or ½ grapefruit, for any fruit listed

To round out your snacks, add some non-starchy vegetables such as celery, carrots, tomatoes, cucumbers, peppers, broccoli, snap peas, and cauliflower.

Snack Ideas
Lower Saturated Fat
25 grams Carbohydrates

- ¾ cup blueberries and skim milk mozzarella cheese
- 1 slice of rice bread and organic sugar-free peanut butter
- 1 nitrate free chicken sausage on a whole grain bun
- *1 medium apple and walnuts
- 1 medium baked potato and low fat cottage cheese
- 2 small corn tortillas, nitrate free turkey, shredded lettuce, tomato, and mayonnaise
- ½ cup hummus, raw carrots/celery, 5 Nut Thin crackers, and almonds
- 1 small raw jicama, chopped and organic sugar-free almond butter
- 1 large whole wheat tortilla, tomatoes, and feta cheese
- 4 cups air popped popcorn and mixed nuts
- *1 large pear and low fat ricotta cheese
- 6 Ak mak crackers and egg, tuna, or chicken salad
- 1½ cups raspberries and low fat cottage cheese
- 2 small corn tortillas, melted skim milk mozzarella, avocado, and fresh salsa
- Hard boiled egg(s) and 1 small grapefruit
- 1¼ cup edemame beans (shelled)

If you have an insulin resistant condition substitute these fruits, ½ cup blueberries, 1 cup other berries or ½ grapefruit, for any fruit listed

To round out your snacks, add some non-starchy vegetables such as celery, carrots, tomatoes, cucumbers, peppers, broccoli, snap peas, and cauliflower.

Step 2: Stress Management, including getting enough sleep

Basic Requirement:

- Eight hours of sleep every night, more if you are very busy or stressed. If you are unable to get eight hours of sleep because of a work schedule, make up for the lost hours when you are not working. However, it is strongly recommended that you get eight hours of uninterrupted sleep every night.
- If you have previously slept less than eight hours a night, you need to make up the hours of sleep you lost by sleeping more than eight hours each night.
- You are required to do two or more Minis (see chapter 6 page 100) a day to help you slow down the breaking down process of every-day life.
- Schedule downtime every day. It is recommended but not required that you do at least one of the following exercises per day. If you don't do these exercises, do something else on a daily basis to rest your brain.

Exercise 1: Relax Those Muscles

Most of us become tense when we are under stress, so it is important to learn to release the tension from your body. Practice the muscle relaxation technique below to ease the effects of a tense day. This exercise is beneficial because it is a way to completely relax your body and put your brain at rest.

- Get comfortable in your favorite chair.
- Breathe deeply and concentrate on your body and how it feels as you sit in the chair. Notice any tension in your neck, shoulders or back.

- Continue breathing and concentrating this way for a few minutes.
- Begin to contract your muscles, starting with your toes and feet; keep your muscles contracted for a few seconds and then slowly relax them. Focus on the feeling of contracting and relaxing your muscles.
- Work your way up your body, continuing to contract and relax your muscles as you go from your feet, to your calves, to your thighs, to your stomach, to your buttocks, to your arms and to your neck—ending with your facial muscles.

When you are finished, take a few more deep breaths. You will notice how much tension you have released and how much better you feel.

Exercise 2: Positive Thinking

Many people get into trouble because they end up thinking and worrying about all the negative things that are happening in their lives. The more you focus on the negative, the worse your situation becomes. Here is a short exercise to help pattern your thought processes to a more positive outlook.

- Find a quiet spot.
- Stop what you are doing and identify what is disturbing you.
- Place your hand over your heart to center your emotions.
- Think of a positive, humorous or joyful event, person or place. For the next few minutes, imagine yourself back in that event, or spending time with that person, or being in that place.
- Next, think of something that you absolutely love and cherish, such as a family member or a beloved pet. Focus on that loving feeling for a few minutes.
- Lastly, reflect on something that you are thankful for in your life.

A big reason for a damaged metabolism is not getting enough sleep or not getting sleep at the right time of the night. Make sure that you get at least 8 hours of uninterrupted sleep a night and that you don't go to bed any later than 11:00 P.M. You will have to make up for any lost sleep in the past before you can consider yourself to not be sleep deprived. You may have to be treated with desyrel, a sleep resetting medication, if you are not sleeping well and the sleep supplements suggested in Chapter Six do not work.

Stress management is theoretically the easiest part of the process since it only involves sleeping and learning to relax. But don't take it for granted! Sometimes sleep and relaxation are easier said than done. If you are having problems in either area, turn to Chapter 6 for tips.

It is Step 2 where you are required to work on all your emotional stresses, too. Seek counseling if needed. You don't have to solve all your issues at once but you must eat well and sleep through the night in order to handle them better.

Notice!

If you are having an unusually difficult time eating and sleeping correctly, or you are eating and sleeping well but are still experiencing problems with mood, energy or chronic health conditions, now is a good time to have your hormone levels checked.

Step 3: Tapering Off Toxic Chemicals or Avoiding Them Completely

Basic Requirement:

- Toxic chemicals should be tapered off and eliminated from worst to best in the specific order listed on the next page.
- Over-the-counter and prescription medication should be tapered

off or changed to a better medication or supplement as soon as possible. (Refer back to chapter 7 for specific recommendations)

This Step is to be addressed after Steps 1, 2 and 5 as needed. You need to eat well, sleep through the night, have any missing hormones balanced before you work on stopping your toxic chemical intake. You use these chemicals to self-medicate natural chemical imbalances. However, you can work on improving the toxic chemicals you ingest and tapering off of sugar as you work on your daily nutrition habits, but never stop sugar before eating well.

I call a chemical toxic if the body cannot use it to rebuild. This includes refined sugars, alcohol, nicotine, artificial sugars, caffeine and many prescription drugs. These substances accelerate the turnover of chemicals and cells in your body, and therefore; speed up the normal aging process.

Up until now, you've been continuing to consume toxic chemicals in order to self-medicate your way through meal planning and stress management. If you have made significant improvements in your nutrition, stress and sleep issues—and hormone issues if needed—it is now time to begin tapering off of all those harmful chemicals one by one. The good news is that now that you are eating properly, relaxing and following a good supplement protocol your body doesn't need all these other stimuli.

Do not try to stop these chemicals before you are ready. You will not heal faster because you stop. Stopping too early will either make it impossible for you to eat correctly or get a good night's rest.

Don't be stoic and automatically assume you can quit these habits cold turkey. And don't try to quit everything at once; switch to a toxic chemical further down the list if it helps you get off a toxic chemical higher on the list. Caffeine is a great substitute for more harmful substances. If you haven't been drinking tea, you may need to start in order to get off of tobacco, alcohol and refined sugars. Never, under any circumstances, go the other way on this list.

If you have skipped directly to this step, stop now! These toxic chemicals—including the consumption of sugar—are not the underlying cause of your weight and health problems, and simply stopping them will not cause you to lose weight or heal your metabolism. You must correct your eating, sleeping, stress and hormone problems first.

Order of Toxic Chemicals, from Worst to Best

Illicit drugs
Tobacco
Alcohol
Artificial sugars
Sugar and sugary foods
Additives, chemical preservatives and other fake chemicals
Caffeine

Illicit Drugs

Stop immediately. If you are using illicit drugs and can't quit, seek professional help.

Tobacco

It is extremely important to get off of tobacco sooner than later, especially if you have heart disease, diabetes, or any vascular disease such as high blood pressure, blood clots or stroke. The first thing to do is get off of tobacco by switching to all nicotine products. The following suggestions can help you eliminate tobacco and nicotine.

- Switch to nicotine patches, inhalers, nasal sprays or gum, and then taper off these nicotine products on a predetermined schedule.

- Decrease the amount of tobacco products you use on a predetermined schedule.
- Try hypnosis, acupuncture or another stop-smoking program.
- Use any of the prescription antismoking medications that contain the chemical bupropion hydrochloride.
- Substitute one stimulating lifestyle habit for another by drinking caffeinated beverages, eating sugary foods or overdoing cardiovascular exercises. Make sure that you get clearance from your physician before you start an exercise program.

NOTE: Make sure that you are taking N-acetyl cysteine, extra vitamin C and vitamin E (mixed tocopherols) while you are still smoking. These supplements will help block some of the damaging effects of tobacco.

Alcohol

Alcohol is a powerful form of self-medication. Make sure to taper off and not stop it cold turkey. Taking GABA before you start drinking for the day or night can lessen your need for alcohol. Taking the 12 supplements recommended in Step 1, especially L-glutamine, will also help alcohol cravings. For women in menopause, getting enough estradiol can help decrease your need for alcohol. If you are alcohol-dependent or have trouble tapering off alcohol using the schedule below, you should consider seeking professional help.

- Start by cutting your alcohol intake in half. If you drink two glasses of wine every night with dinner, taper off to one glass of wine. If you drink eight beers with your friends on a weekend night, cut back to four beers. *There is no room for hard liquor on this program.* If you are using it, switch to red wine or beer.
- Continue tapering off your intake by one-half at a pace you are comfortable with, but preferably make at least one change every two weeks.

Artificial Sugars

Stop all artificial sugars cold turkey. Use stevia or xylitol if needed, or switch to organic raw honey or blackstrap molasses (as long as you do not have an insulin resistant condition) and taper off that at your own pace. In general, refined sugars are better than artificial sugars. Get off of diet sodas by either drinking caffeinated teas or coffee or by switching to caffeinated waters.

Sugar and Sugary Foods

Remember that your ultimate goal is to taper off refined sugar products entirely. As impossible as this may sound right now, as you heal your metabolism your sweet tooth will go away. If you need to continue refined sugar for a while, organic raw honey or blackstrap molasses are the best kinds to use. Or you could try small amounts of Stevia or xylitol.

Do *not* skip your balanced meals or snacks—and do not substitute sugary foods for balanced meals. Instead, use the following suggestions if you have sugar cravings.

If you have extreme sugar cravings:

- Give in to your craving early to avoid greater cravings later on.
- Try to eat high glycemic index fruits with a protein source or dark unsweetened chocolate.
- If this doesn't satisfy you, have one dessert made from natural ingredients and whole fat. (This is not an endorsement to overeat desserts.) Do not have candy or sodas.

If you have mild sugar cravings

- Eat fruits with the lowest glycemic index together with a protein source.

- Switch from caffeinated sodas to caffeinated coffee or tea with liquid Stevia or small amounts of organic raw honey. Switch decaffeinated sodas to herbal teas or fruit flavored waters.

Additives, Chemical Preservatives and Other Fake Chemicals

If you have not already stopped eating packaged and processed foods, now is the time to do so. There is no need to taper down your consumption of preservatives, additives, MSG, fake fats or carbohydrate and fat blockers. Stop them cold turkey.

Caffeine

Caffeine is the least harmful of the toxic chemicals. You may need to continue a cup or two of coffee or tea for a very long time. However, it is important that you wean yourself down to this amount in order to fully heal. Go slowly. Try weaning yourself off caffeinated beverages by switching from the worst sources (diet sodas) to the best sources (green tea) in this order:

Diet sodas
Sodas
Caffeinated waters
Yerba Mate
Coffee
Black tea
Green tea

Try this method to help wean yourself down:

Start by switching to 3/4 caffeine and 1/4 decaffeinated for each caffeinated beverage you normally consume. Do not taper off the number of beverages that you drink in a day. If you do not feel any ill

effects after a week, cut back to 1/2 caffeine and 1/2 decaffeinated for each beverage. After a week, assuming you feel okay, taper off to ¼ caffeine and ¾ decaffeinated for each beverage. You could be completely off the caffeinated form of this beverage by the fourth week. If you feel lousy after cutting back your caffeine intake at any point, try to continue on this amount of caffeine for another week and re-evaluate how you feel. If this doesn't work, resume the same amount of caffeine as the prior week or switch to caffeinated coffee or tea. If you have to start over, do not despair. This is perfectly normal. You will get there. Do this until you are drinking one to two cups of coffee or tea a day. Then go on to another issue and revisit coming fully off of caffeine another day, month or year.

> *By this time you should be drinking plenty of water to substitute for all the sodas, juices, milk and caffeinated drinks that you have stopped drinking.*

Over-the-Counter Drugs

Once you have worked on the underlying reason you are using these drugs, you should be able to get off your over-the-counter drugs without any harmful effects. So stop them one by one and gauge the reaction or simply switch over to the suggestions found in Chapter 7. Stop over-the-counter drugs immediately if you realize you are using them to treat an annoying symptom such as a stuffy nose when you get a cold.

Prescription Drugs

If you are taking prescription drugs, discuss with your physician the option of stopping or lowering the dose or switching to another medicine with fewer side effects. (Refer to Chapter 7 for more details.)

Please remember to always consult your physician when changing your intake of prescription drugs.

Step 4: Smart Exercise

Basic Requirement:

Up to three days a week of strenuous exercise with additional nonstrenuous exercise as follows:

- Three nonconsecutive days: 30 to 45 minutes of adaptive exercise with stretching.
- Two days, other than the adaptive exercise days: 30 minutes of . calming exercises.
- No stimulating exercises, unless for self-medication.
- You can add calming exercises for the other two days of the week if you so desire, but it is recommended that you rest if you have a very damaged metabolism.

Only those with a healthy metabolism should cross train. If you have a damaged metabolism, stimulating exercises will make you worse in the long term. Stop doing them until your metabolism has healed. Here are the acceptable exercises for the Healing Plan. By doing more adaptive and calming, you give your body the chance to catch up on rebuilding. Stimulating exercises break you down.

Acceptable Adaptive Exercises:

- Ball and band work
- Core strength exercises/mat classes/calisthenics
- Light weight routine
- Pilates
- Pool exercises
- Yoga (strengthening types of yoga only)

Acceptable Calming Exercises:

- Light stretching
- Restorative yoga (not Bikhram)
- Tai chi or other similar martial arts practices
- Slow swimming*
- Slow walking*

Only calming if you keep your heart rate at or below 90 beats a minute the whole time.

Unacceptable Stimulating Exercises:

- Aerobic machines
- Aerobics classes
- Bikhram yoga
- Fast biking
- Fast swimming
- Fast walking/hiking
- Kickboxing
- Running/jogging
- Similar stimulating exercises and activities not listed here
- Soccer, tennis, volleyball or other vigorous sports
- Spinning exercise bike classes
- Weight lifting (heavy)

If you have skipped directly to this step, stop now! Simply starting or changing your exercise routine will not solve your weight or health issues. You must correct your eating, sleeping, stress and hormone problems first. An exception is if you need to completely stop all exercise because it is causing you to be emotionally or physically fatigued.

If you are exercising more than recommended or have not been exercising at all, don't try to match the workout requirement the first day. Follow the appropriate instructions below to help your body adjust to your new routine.

Starting an Exercise Routine

If you are out of shape and over the age of 50, consult your physician for clearance to exercise. If you have multiple health problems, consider starting your program at an exercise rehabilitation center. Your physician can advise you about facilities in your area. If you have back, neck or joint problems, always consult your physician before starting any exercise routine.

If you have not been exercising at all, use the adaptive and calming exercises I laid out in Chapter 8. Begin by choosing three exercises from the adaptive program and two from the calming program, doing 8 to 12 repetitions of each one. Do this program three times a week, resting one day between each session. Within two to four weeks, you should be able to work up to doing 8 to 12 repetitions of all 10 exercises, three times a week.

As your energy improves, add slow walking or one of the other acceptable calming exercises for half an hour, two times a week, on the days that you are not doing your adaptive workout. You may also vary your adaptive workout, but *don't try to do more than the recommended total amount of exercise.* You are not going to improve your metabolism or decrease the amount of fat weight gain you will experience during your transition if you exercise when you are mentally or physically exhausted. Don't push it. Exercising too early on in the healing process will slow your healing!

> *Do not use this program as an excuse to never exercise. A moderate exercise program is an integral part of the Schwarzbein Principle Program. It just needs to be introduced at the right time and in the right way to be beneficial.*

If you are interested in working out with me in the privacy of your own home, check out my exercise videos at *www.schwarzbeinprinciple.com.*

Tapering Off of Overexercising

If you are overexercising as a form of self-medication, you need to taper down the amount of stimulating exercises you are doing to a reasonable amount. Decrease the length of your workout by 15 minutes a day every week until you are only exercising 30 minutes a day. Then switch to working out 30 minutes every other day with slow walking for the 30 minutes on the days in between. You can stay at 30 minutes every other day if you are not getting exhausted from your exercise routine. However, it is preferable that you switch to an adaptive exercise routine or taper completely off of stimulating exercises by decreasing to 15 minutes every other day for a week and then stopping altogether the next week. If you feel you can stop stimulating exercises on a faster schedule without falling apart mentally and physically, by all means do so.

When your metabolism has healed and you are following the Maintenance Plan, you may begin doing stimulating exercises again, but remember—*you never have to do any stimulating exercises ever again to have a long, healthy and heart-disease free life or your ideal body composition.*

Step 5: Hormone Replacement Therapy, as needed

Fixing your hormone issue is the only way to achieve true balance. The only way to know if you have a hormone problem is to have your levels checked. You cannot do this one on your own. Please review Chapter 9 if you know or think you may have a hormone problem. Work with a health professional who understands that all hormone systems are interconnected and that one hormone out of balance means that all your hormones are out of balance.

Graduating to the Maintenance Plan

Once you have completed all five steps of the Schwarzbein Program Healing Plan, retake the metabolism quiz on page 183.

If you do not pass the quiz, you still have a damaged metabolism and will need to continue following the Healing Plan guidelines. Do not be discouraged! It takes time to heal, but it's well worth the effort. I applaud you for getting this far and congratulate you for making all the necessary changes to your nutrition and lifestyle habits. It is now only a matter or time. Retake the quiz when you are ready and when you pass move on to the Maintenance Plan.

If you pass the quiz, you have healed your metabolism. I also applaud you for getting this far and congratulate you for all the positive changes you have made. If you passed the first time around, your metabolism wasn't as damaged as you may have thought. You are now entering the next phase of the SPP. It is at this stage that you can finish burning off any excess fat weight, if needed. It is time to move on to the Maintenance Plan.

Thirteen

The Maintenance Plan

The Schwarzbein Principle Program (SPP) Maintenance Plan has been specifically designed to keep your metabolism healthy through making positive changes to your nutrition and lifestyle habits. This plan is for those of you who already have a healthy metabolism or have just healed it. There is no healing phase when you are following this plan, so if you need to repair your metabolism, you need to follow the Healing Plan.

As there is no healing phase in the Maintenance Plan, your body should respond quickly to the lifestyle changes you make, including dramatic weight loss if needed for your body to function at its optimal level. If your body does not respond quickly and you are still experiencing low moods or other physiological problems, have your hormones checked by a professional. Remember, no matter what your lifestyle, you cannot be truly healthy until your hormones are replaced correctly.

If you have recently completed the Healing Plan, a good portion of the material in this chapter will be similar to the material you have already read. *Read it carefully anyway.* There are subtle but important changes between my two plans, and of course it's always a good idea

to have a refresher course in your Schwarzbein lifestyle. In fact, even after you have completed the Maintenance Plan, I suggest you re-read this chapter periodically to make sure you are truly getting the maximum benefits from the program.

Remember to follow these steps in the order you determined in your personal assessment. If you skip ahead, you will not get the full benefits of the program.

Step 1: Healthy Nutrition, including taking supplements if needed

Basic Requirement:

- Eat four "squares" of quality protein, real carbohydrates, healthy fats, and nonstarchy vegetables a day; three meals and at least one snack. If you need to lose weight or you find yourself gaining weight by eating four times a day, spread your food out and eat smaller portions five or more times a day and follow the low saturated fat guidelines.
- Do *not* skip meals or count calories. This is not a low-calorie diet.
- Follow the prescribed eating requirements for each food group.
- Use the four supplements listed on page 84 on a daily basis (recommended, not required).

The SPP maintenance plan *encourages* you to eat smaller portions more frequently, but it is not a low-calorie diet. On this plan, you will be eating plenty of food, just spreading it out more evenly.

Do not skip meals or snacks. I understand that making the time to eat more frequently can be hard to do, but this is one of the most important things you will be doing for yourself on a daily basis.

Refer to the food lists in Chapter 5: Nutrition for acceptable foods in each category.

Protein Requirements:

Men:
- 13 to 23 ounces per day:
  3 to 5 ounces (21 to 35 grams) with meals; 2 to 4 ounces (14 to 28 grams) with snacks.

Women:
- 8 to 18 ounces per day:
  2 to 4 ounces (14 to 28 grams) with meals; 1 to 3 ounces (7 to 21 grams) with snacks.

It is also acceptable to divide the total ounces evenly between the four meal times.

The taller you are, the more you weigh and the more active you are, the higher your protein needs.

Protein Requirement Calculations

If you wish, you can calculate protein requirements for your specific sex, body type and activity level by following the instructions provided in Appendix A.

Quality Protein Portions

You can approximate your protein portion requirement by sight. One ounce of protein is approximately ¼ the size of your palm and as thick as a deck of a cards. The food equivalent is:

1 ounce ground sirloin, cuts of lamb, pork, chicken, meat, turkey and fish

1 egg

1 ounce canned tuna (⅙ of can)

¼ cup organic cottage cheese

1 ounce organic whole milk mozzarella or feta cheese

⅜ cup tofu

¼ cup tempeh

Nuts: ⅛ cup soybeans, 1ounce almonds, 1½ ounce other nuts

Use these quantities to determine the amount you should eat for each protein portion. For instance, if you want to eat three ounces of protein, simply multiply the portions above by three.

Carbohydrate Requirements:

- Four sittings: 150 grams of carbohydrates per day; 40 grams per meal and 30 grams per snack.
- Five sittings: 150 grams of carbohydrates per day, 30 grams per sitting.
- If you are Extremely Active (see Appendix A, page 256): 200 grams of carbohydrates per day, 50 per four sittings or 40 per five sittings, until you taper down to Very Active and then eat 175 grams of carbohydrates per day, approximately 45 per four sittings and 35 per five sittings.
- Fruit: No more than three servings per day. Count your fruit serving as a carbohydrate when you eat it as a snack and as a free

food when you eat it as part of your meal. This will ensure that you get plenty of complex carbohydrates and not just refined sugars in a day.

- For fat weight loss: Eat no more than one serving of fruit a day, preferably from the low glycemic index.

If you are appalled at the "high" amount of carbohydrates per meal, you have succumbed to the false promises of one of the popular diets promoting too few carbohydrates. If you don't eat enough carbohydrates, you send signals to your body that it is in the middle of a famine causing your body to "eat" its own lean muscle tissue for energy. Decreasing your carbohydrate intake causes "starvation" weight loss at first, but increases the probability that you will gain fat weight in the long term.

Fat Requirements:
- Plenty of monounsaturated and natural saturated fats.
- Small amounts of polyunsaturated fats.
- Avoid all damaged fats (transfatty acids, rancid fats, partially hydrogenated oils and fully hydrogenated oils).
- For fat weight loss: less than three grams of long-chain natural saturated fat per sitting.

Nonstarchy Vegetable Requirements:
- Minimum of one cup serving at every meal, half cup at snacks.

Don't be shy about nonstarchy vegetables. The more you eat, the better. Do not count these as carbohydrates. A nonstarchy vegetable is any portion of a half cup that contains five grams or less of

carbohydrate. Make sure that you are eating a variety of nonstarchy vegetables and not the same ones each time, otherwise you won't get all the benefits from the different plant chemicals.

Supplement Requirements

It is highly recommended *but not required* that you take all of the following supplements to keep your metabolism healthy:

- A good twice-a-day multivitamin and mineral.
- High quality omega-3 fish oils.
- Stress B complex.
- Calcium and magnesium added at bedtime.

These four supplements are what I generally recommend for maintenance. Unfortunately, they are not always enough if you have a very busy lifestyle. Consider adding some of the supplements listed in Chapter 5 if you feel you need additional help.

Six Helpful Hints to Changing Food Habits

1. Do not invite the enemy to the table
- If you are served a breadbasket, ask the waitperson to remove it from the table.
- Don't order foods you should not be eating such as pizza and pasta dishes.
- Don't keep bad food choices stocked at home. In fact this is a great time to go through your cupboards and clean out all the "non-foods" that are not on this plan
- Ask your friends and family to be courteous and not flaunt your favorite junk food in your face or eat it when you are around.

Six Helpful Hints to Changing Food Habits (cont'd)

2. The 3-bite rule for special occasions

- If you feel that you must have something on a special occasion that is not on your plan follow the 3-bite rule and only have three small bites. This is not the same as when you give in to an out-of-control craving.

3. Speak up when dining at someone's home

- Start by asking them what they are making so you know whether or not you will be able to eat it. Then, depending on your level of comfort, ask them to make you something different if it doesn't fit your plan or bring your own food. Once my friends and family knew what I expected to be fed, they would plan a healthy meal around the things that I could eat. This way all the other guests got a healthier meal, too!

4. Don't feel guilty if you are not perfect

- The changes you are making take time. This is a process. I guarantee you will not be able to be perfect all the time. But if you concentrate on not skipping meals and eating balanced meals, I give you my word that eating this way will get easier and easier until you no longer have to think about it.

5. Think ahead when traveling or at work

- It is guaranteed that you will not get served real food when you travel. Take mixed nuts with or without raisins for snacks and bring food from home to eat on the plane.
- Buy yourself a cooler and keep staple foods in it for when you are traveling in the car.
- At work, stock the company refrigerator with healthy foods and bring your lunch with you.

6. Journal your food, mood and exercise intake.

It has been shown that keeping a food and lifestyle journal helps keep you accountable and helps you make changes to your habits faster and permanently. You can download food, mood and exercise diary sheets off my website at *http://www.schwarzbeinprinciple.com/pgs/dr_schw/institute1.html* or create your own.

Meal Plans

Create your own meal plans by following these four recommendations or follow the predesigned meal plans starting on page 233:

1 Choose a quality protein—with or without significant amounts of long chain saturated fats.
2. Include real carbohydrates.
3. Eat a variety of nonstarchy vegetables throughout the day, as much as you like.
4. Add healthy fats in moderate amounts.

Use the meal plans as a template for formulating your own meal plans. Remember to rotate your foods and eat a variety of different choices to obtain beneficial nutrients and to avoid food allergies. I have included a 30-gram gluten free meal plan here in case you need to follow a gluten free diet. For more information on food allergies see Appendix B or visit my Web site at *www.schwarzbeinprinciple.com.*

30 gram Sample Menu Plan

Each meal contains approximately 30 grams of carbohydrates

MEALS	MONDAY	TUESDAY	WEDNESDAY	THURSDAY	FRIDAY	SATURDAY	SUNDAY
Breakfast	1/2 cup cottage cheese w/ 1 peach, chopped 1 piece toast w/butter mixed raw nuts *raw veggies	Veggie Omelet w/spinach, mushrooms, and peppers 1 cup roasted potatoes	Breakfast Burrito: eggs, mozzarella cheese, avocado, and tomato wrapped in a large corn tortilla	Turkey sausage 1 cup oatmeal w/1/2 cup mixed berries and crushed walnuts *carrot sticks	Organic sugar-free almond butter on 2 slices of whole wheat sprouted bread hard boiled egg 1/2 medium jicama, chopped *raw veggies	1 cup plain whole milk yogurt mixed w/1/2 cup blueberries and slivered almonds celery and organic sugar-free peanut butter	2 eggs, over easy 1 slice toast w/ butter 1 small orange *cherry tomatoes
Lunch	Burger w/sautéed mushrooms and swiss cheese on 2 pieces whole grain bread, lettuce, tomato, onion, dijon & pure pressed oil mayonnaise	Grilled shrimp, salmon, or chicken Caesar salad, no croutons, Newman's Caesar dressing 8 Edward & Son rice snaps 1 small apple	New England Clam Chowder (heavy organic whipping cream) 3 Ak Mak crackers 1/4 cup hummus w/carrots, celery, and peppers	Southwest Salad: mixed greens, grilled seasoned chicken or sirloin, 1/2 cup corn, 1/3 cup black beans, fresh salsa, and guacamole	1/2 baked potato w/ mozzarella cheese and broccoli florets 3/4 cup unshelled edamame (soy beans)	Tuna salad made w/ pure pressed oil mayonnaise on mixed greens, cherry tomatoes, and red onions 3 Wasa hearty rye crispbread	Chicken sandwich: grilled chicken breast, feta crumbles, lettuce, tomato, onion, and pesto basil mayo (made w/pure-pressed oil) on 2 slices whole grain bread
Dinner	Grilled, lightly blackened Red Snapper 1 cup butternut squash 1/3 cup couscous Mixed green salad w/ vinaigrette	Roasted pork loin 1 medium potato w/ butter & chives Steamed broccoli and cauliflower Tomato, mozzarella, and basil salad w/ balsamic vinaigrette	Fish/shrimp/chix tacos: 2 corn tortillas, fish of choice or shrimp or chicken, diced cabbage, tomato, and avocado served with fresh salsa and squeezed lemon Add salad if desired	Grilled seasoned tofu or chicken 1/2 cup brown rice 1/4 cup lentils Roasted red peppers and steamed snap peas Add salad if desired	Roasted turkey 1 large steamed artichoke w/ pure pressed oil mayo 1/2 medium sweet potato Mixed green salad w/Annie's Italian dressing	Beef or chicken kabobs w/peppers, onion & mushrooms 2/3 cup brown rice Small Caesar salad, no croutons, Newman's caesar dressing	Grilled salmon Corn on the cob, 1 ear Sautéed spinach, garlic, and olive oil Mixed green salad w/vinaigrette

1. When bread is indicated, use: Ezekial, Vogel or Alvarado; Crackers: AkMak, Lavosh, Wasa, Edward & Son (brown rice snaps), 365 Woven Wheats
2. Pitas: Cedarlane; Tortillas: Corn, Alvarado Street; Dressings: Drew's, Spectrum, Newman's Own Oil & Vinegar and Caesar, Annie's Italian
3. If raw vegetables are indicated, use: carrots, celery, onions, cucumber, broccoli, cauliflower, peppers, Mixed greens could include: variety of lettuce, spinach, onions, tomatoes, grated carrots, cucumber, celery, peppers.
4. When butter is indicated, use organic, unsweetened, unsalted butter.

30 gram Gluten Free Sample Menu Plan

*Each meal contains approximately **30 grams** of carbohydrates*

MEALS	MONDAY	TUESDAY	WEDNESDAY	THURSDAY	FRIDAY	SATURDAY	SUNDAY
Breakfast	Burrito: Eggs, muenster cheese, avocado slices, chopped tomato wrapped in a large corn tortilla	1 1/4 cup cream of rice w/cinnamon and crushed walnuts String cheese *Carrot sticks	Scoop of eggless egg salad (made from tofu) on Nut Thins (20 crackers) *Sliced tomatoes	Scrambled eggs Fresh salsa 1/3 cup black beans 1 small corn tortilla	Cottage cheese 1 slice rice bread toast w/organic sugar-free almond butter *raw veggies	Hard boiled egg(s) 1 1/4cup hot amaranth cereal Celery dipped in natural peanut butter	Vegetable scramble Eggs, broccoli, onions, spinach, and feta cheese 1 cup roasted potatoes
Lunch	1 medium baked potato stuffed w/1/2 cup cottage cheese and steamed broccoli	Mexican salad: Lettuce, seasoned ground sirloin, 1/3 cup kidney beans, 1/2 cup corn, fresh salsa, and guacamole	1 cup plain whole milk yogurt 2 cups air popped popcorn + mixed nuts raw veggies	Scoop of tuna salad (made with chopped onions, celery, and pure oil pressed mayo) 16 Edward & Son brown rice snaps	Grilled salmon Cold bean salad: black beans, kidney beans, corn, tomato, cilantro, garlic, and olive oil tossed together: 3/4 cup portion	Chinese chicken salad: mixed greens, shredded cabbage, grilled chicken, and almond slivers Oriental dressing (no sugar) 1 small/medium jicama, chopped	Turkey sandwich: 1 slice rice bread, nitrate free turkey, lettuce, tomato, onions, pure pressed oil mayonnaise
Dinner	Grilled lamb chops 3/4 cup brown rice Grilled zucchini Mixed greens salad w/vinaigrette	Grilled salmon 1/2 c red potatoes 1/2 c corn Sautéed spinach Chopped cucumber, carrots and tomatoes w/vinaigrette	Stir-fried pork and vegetables served over 2/3 cup buckwheat Add salad if desired	Baked halibut 1 medium sweet potato w/a dab of butter Mixed green salad w/ vinaigrette	Grilled chicken 1 large artichoke, steamed Broccoli and cauliflower mix Add salad if desired	Tuna Melt: Tuna salad made with pure pressed oil, lettuce, thick slice of tomato, and melted mozzarella on 1 sl rice bread Mixed green salad w/vinaigrette	Steak smothered with sautéed onions, mushrooms, and peppers Medium baked potato w/a dab of butter Small Caesar salad, Newman's Caesar dressing, no croutons

1. When bread is indicated, use: Rice Bread; Crackers: Edward & Son (brown rice snaps), Nut Thins, Black Sesame Seed Rice Crackers (Whole Foods); Tortillas: Corn Dressings: Drew's, Spectrum, Newman's Own Oil & Vinegar and Caesar, Annie's Italian

2. If raw vegetables are indicated, use: carrots, celery, onions, cucumber, broccoli, cauliflower, peppers.

3. Mixed greens could include: variety of lettuce, spinach, onions, tomatoes, grated carrots, cucumber, celery, peppers.

4. When butter is indicated, use organic, unsweetened, unsalted butter.

40 Gram Sample Menu Plan

Each meal contains approximately 40 grams of carbohydrates

MEALS	MONDAY	TUESDAY	WEDNESDAY	THURSDAY	FRIDAY	SATURDAY	SUNDAY
Breakfast	Scrambled eggs with onions & spinach 1 small corn tortilla 1 cup oatmeal w/organic whipping cream	Breakfast sandwich: Scrambled eggs, nitrite free ham, muenster cheese, and sliced tomato on 2 slices Ezekial toast 1/4 medium jicama, chopped	Scoop of eggless egg salad (made w/ tofu) on 10 Ak mak crackers Celery and organic sugar-free peanut butter	Hard boiled eggs Organic, sugar-free almond butter on 2 slices Vogel toast 1/2 cup cream of rice cereal w/ butter and cinnamon *carrot sticks	Nitrate-free turkey sausage(s) 1 1/3 cup roasted potatoes w/ onions and peppers *Sliced tomatoes	Scrambled eggs 2 small corn tortillas 1/4 cup black beans Fresh salsa *Raw veggies	2 slices of sprouted wheat bread w/organic, sugar-free peanut butter Cottage cheese 2/3 cup butternut squash w/ cinnamon *carrot sticks
Lunch	Grilled chicken on mixed greens with 1/3 cup corn, 1/3 cup chick peas, 1/3 cup kidney beans, cucumber, cherry tomatoes, and goat cheese crumbles w/ vinaigrette	2 fish tacos: Broiled fish of choice on 2 small corn tortillas w/ shredded cabbage, 1/4 cup beans, avocado slices, fresh salsa, and a dab of sour cream	Turkey burger w/ sautéed mushrooms and swiss cheese on 2 pieces whole grain bread, lettuce, tomato, onion, dijon & pure pressed oil mayonnaise 1 1/2 cups air-popped popcorn	Tuna salad made w/ pure pressed oil mayonnaise on mixed greens, cherry tomatoes, and red onions 5 Wasa hearty rye crispbreads	Grilled shrimp served on a bed of romaine w/ feta cheese crumbles, tomato wedges, green onions, and snap peas served w/ vinaigrette 3/4 cup lentil or bean soup	Chicken soup (without noodles) 3 Ak Mak crackers 1/2 cup hummus w/ carrots, celery, and peppers	Grilled shrimp, salmon, or chicken Caesar salad, no croutons, Newman's Caesar dressing 12 Edward & Son rice snaps 1/2 medium jicama, chopped
Dinner	Grilled seasoned tofu or chicken 3/4cup tabouleh Roasted red peppers and steamed snap peas Add salad if desired	Grilled lamb chops Green beans 1 medium/large sweet potato w/butter Small Caesar salad, no croutons, Newman's ceasar dressing	Sirloin steak Corn on the cob, 1 small ear w/butter 1/2 cup brown rice Sauteed spinach, garlic, and olive oil Mixed green salad w/vinaigrette	Grilled chicken kabobs w/ peppers, onions, and mushrooms 3/4 cup couscous Tomato, mozzarella, and basil salad w/ balsamic vinaigrette	Stir-fried pork and vegetables 3/4 cup buckwheat Mixed green salad w/Annie's Italian	Grilled sea bass 3/4 cup wild rice Mushroom caps sautéed in garlic and olive oil Chopped carrots, cucumber, and tomatoes w/ vinaigrette	NY Steak 3/4 cup quinoa Asparagus spears Mixed green salad w/vinaigrette

1. When bread is indicated, use: Ezekial, Vogel or Alvarado Crackers: AkMak, Lavosh, Wasa, Edward & Son (brown rice snaps), 365 Woven Wheats Pitas: Cedarlane Tortillas: Corn, Alvarado Street Dressings: Drew's, Spectrum, Newman's Own Oil & Vinegar and Caesar, Annie's Italian
2. If raw vegetables are indicated, use: carrots, celery, onions, cucumber, broccoli, cauliflower, peppers
3. Mixed greens could include: variety of lettuce, spinach, onions, tomatoes, grated carrots, cucumber, celery, peppers.
4. When butter is indicated, use organic, raw unsweetened, unsalted butter.

40 Gram Low Saturated Fat Sample Menu Plan

Each meal contains approximately 40 grams of carbohydrates

MEALS	MONDAY	TUESDAY	WEDNESDAY	THURSDAY	FRIDAY	SATURDAY	SUNDAY
Breakfast	Scrambled eggs with onions & spinach 1 small corn tortilla 1 cup oatmeal	Breakfast sandwich: Scrambled eggs, nitrite free ham, skim milk mozz cheese, and sliced tomato on 2 slices Ezekial toast 1/4 medium jicama, chopped	Scoop of eggless egg salad (made w/ tofu) on 10 Ak Mak crackers Celery and organic sugar-free peanut butter	Hard boiled eggs Organic, sugar-free almond butter on 2 slices Vogel toast 1/2 cup cream of rice cereal w/cinnamon *carrot sticks	Nitrate-free turkey sausage(s) 1 1/3 cup roasted potatoes w/onions and peppers *Sliced tomatoes	Scrambled eggs 2 small corn tortillas 1/4 cup black beans Fresh salsa *Raw veggies	2 slices of sprouted whole grain bread w/organic, sugar-free peanut butter Low fat cottage cheese 2/3 cup butternut squash w/ cinnamon *carrot sticks
Lunch	Grilled chicken on mixed greens with 1/3 cup corn, 1/3 cup chick peas, 1/3 cup kidney beans, cucumber, and cherry tomatoes w/ vinaigrette	2 fish tacos: Broiled fish of choice on 2 small corn tortillas w/ shredded cabbage, 1/4 cup beans, avocado slices, and fresh salsa	Turkey burger w/ sautéed mushrooms on 2 pieces whole grain bread, lettuce, tomato, onion, dijon & pure pressed oil mayonnaise 1 1/2 cups air popped popcorn	Tuna salad made w/ pure pressed oil mayonnaise on mixed greens, cherry tomatoes, and red onions 5 Wasa hearty rye crispbreads	Grilled shrimp served on a bed of romaine w/tomato wedges, green onions, and snap peas served w/vinaigrette 3/4 cup lentil or bean soup	Chicken soup (no noodles) 3 Ak Mak crackers 1/2 cup hummus w/carrots, celery, and peppers	Grilled shrimp, salmon, or chicken Caesar salad, no croutons, Newman's Caesar dressing 12 Edward & Son rice snaps 1/2 medium jicama, chopped
Dinner	Grilled seasoned tofu or chicken 3/4 cup tabouleh Roasted red peppers and steamed snap peas Add salad if desired	Grilled lamb chops Green beans 1 medium/large sweet potato w/a dab of butter Small Caesar salad, no croutons, Newman's caesar dressing	Sirloin steak Corn on the cob, 1 small ear 1/2 cup brown rice Sautéed spinach, garlic, and olive oil Mixed green salad w/ vinaigrette	Grilled chicken kabobs w/ peppers, onions, and mushrooms 3/4 cup couscous Tomato, mozzarella, and basil salad w/balsamic vinaigrette	Stir-fried pork and vegetables 3/4 cup buckwheat Mixed green salad w/ Annie's Italian	Grilled sea bass 3/4 cup wild rice Mushroom caps sautéed in garlic and olive oil Chopped carrots, cucumber, and tomatoes w/vinaigrette	Cornish Hen 3/4 cup quinoa Asparagus spears Mixed green salad w/vinaigrette

1. When bread is indicated, use: Ezekial, Vogel or Alvarado; Crackers: AkMak, Lavosh, Wasa, Edward & Son (brown rice snaps), 365 Woven Wheats, Nut Pitas: Cedarlane; Tortillas: Corn, Alvarado Street; Dressings: Drew's, Spectrum, Newman's Own Oil & Vinegar and Caesar, Annie's Italian
2. If raw vegetables are indicated, use: carrots, celery, onions, cucumber, broccoli, cauliflower, peppers.
3. Mixed greens could include: variety of lettuce, spinach, onions, tomatoes, grated carrots, cucumber, celery, peppers.
4. When butter is indicated, use organic, unsweetened, unsalted butter.

Snack Ideas
Regular Diet
30 grams Carbohydrates

- 1 large apple and 2 Tbs. organic sugar-free peanut butter
- 1 medium baked potato and ½ cup cottage cheese
- 1 slice Ezekial bread with sliced avocado, chicken salad and ½ orange
- Muenster cheese, 7 Ak Mak crackers, and spicy mustard
- 1 cup organic, plain, whole milk yogurt, 1 cup strawberries, and mixed nuts
- 2 small corn tortillas, melted mozzarella cheese, sliced avocado, and tomato
- 7 Ak Mak crackers and egg, tuna, or chicken salad
- 1 large pear and goat cheese
- 1 corn tortilla wrapped around ⅓ cup beans/corn & shredded chicken
- 2 brown rice cakes and organic sugar-free cashew butter
- ¾ cup unsweetened applesauce and cottage cheese
- 1 nitrate-free turkey or chicken sausage on a whole grain bun
- 1½ cup fresh pineapple and ricotta cheese
- ½ cup hummus with raw vegetables and almonds
- 1½ cup edamame beans (shelled)

To round out your snacks, add some non-starchy vegetables such as celery, carrots, tomatoes, cucumbers, peppers, broccoli, snap peas, and cauliflower.

Snack Ideas
Lower Saturated Fat
30 grams Carbohydrates

- *1 large apple and organic, sugar-free peanut butter
- 1 medium sweet potato and low-fat cottage cheese
- *1 slice Ezeckial bread with sliced avocado, chicken salad, and 1/2 orange
- 7 Ak Mak crackers, skim milk mozzarella cheese, and spicy mustard
- 1 cup organic, plain, reduced-fat yogurt, 1 cup strawberries, and crushed walnuts
- 23 Nut Thin crackers with egg salad, tuna salad, or chicken salad
- *1 large pear and goat cheese
- 1 corn tortilla wrapped around ⅓ cup pinto beans & shredded chicken
- 1 slice of rice bread and organic, sugar-free cashew butter
- *¾ cup unsweetened applesauce and cottage cheese
- 2 small corn tortillas, melted skim milk mozzarella cheese, sliced avocado, and fresh salsa
- *1½ cup fresh pineapple and ricotta cheese
- ½ cup hummus with raw vegetables, 10 Nut Thin crackers, and almonds
- 1½ cups edamame beans (shelled)

To round out your snacks, add some non-starchy vegetables such as celery, carrots, tomatoes, cucumbers, peppers, broccoli, snap peas, and cauliflower.

———————

*If following the Healing Plan: Substitute ½ cup blueberries, 1 cup other berries, or ½ grapefruit for the fruits listed.

Snack Ideas
Gluten-Free
30 grams Carbohydrates

- 2 cups whole strawberries and ricotta cheese
- 2 slices of gluten free bread (25g) and organic sugar-free peanut butter
- 6 Corn Thins with egg salad, tuna salad, or chicken salad
- 1 medium baked potato with mozzarella cheese and fresh salsa
- 4½ cups air popped popcorn and mixed nuts
- 1½ cup blackberries and sunflower seeds
- 1 slice rice, buckwheat, or millet bread with avocado, and chicken salad
- 1 cup organic, plain, whole milk yogurt, ½ cup blueberries, and crushed walnuts
- 2 slices of gluten free bread (25g), tomatoes, feta cheese, and carrot sticks
- 23 Nut Thin crackers with almond butter
- 1 slice rice bread (30g), nitrate free turkey, lettuce, tomato, and mayonnaise (pure pressed oils)
- 1 medium sweet potato and nitrate free chicken sausage
- 23 Nut Thin crackers, mozzarella cheese and spicy mustard
- 16 Edward & Son brown rice snaps, cucumber, and goat cheese
- 2 small corn tortillas (30g), melted mozzarella cheese, avocado, and fresh salsa
- 1 medium grapefruit and hard boiled egg(s)
- ½ cup hummus, 10 Nut Thin crackers, raw vegetables, and cashews
- 1 cup blueberries and cottage cheese
- 1½ cup edemame beans (shelled)

If following the lower saturated fat guidelines: Substitute part-skim mozzarella, low-fat ricotta, low-fat cottage cheese, or reduced fat plain yogurt for any dairy product listed. Eat limited amounts of sausage.

To round out your snacks, add some non-starchy vegetables such as celery, carrots, tomatoes, cucumbers, peppers, broccoli, snap peas, and cauliflower.

It should take approximately two to four weeks to make the necessary changes to your meal plans including drinking enough water. Sometimes it takes less, and sometimes it takes longer. Remember that this is your personal transition process and you should make the necessary changes to your health as quickly or as slowly as necessary to make this a permanent lifestyle modification.

If you find that you are having a difficult time making the necessary changes, I highly recommend that you take the suggested supplements, and if that doesn't help, that you work with a food coach or dietitian for accountability and suggestions. Or consider that stress or hormone problems may be keeping you from making these changes.

Step 2: Stress Management, including getting enough sleep

Basic Requirement:

- Eight hours of sleep every night, more if you are very busy or stressed. If you are unable to get eight hours of sleep because of a work schedule, make up for the lost hours when you are not working. However, it is strongly recommended that you get eight hours of uninterrupted sleep every night.
- If you have previously slept less than eight hours a night, you need to make up the hours of sleep you lost by sleeping more than eight hours each night.
- You are required to do two or more Minis (see chapter 6 page 100) a day to help you slow down the breaking down process of everyday life.
- Schedule downtime every day. It is recommended but not required that you do at least one of the following exercises per day. If you don't do these exercises, do something else on a daily basis to rest your brain.

Exercise 1: Relax Those Muscles

Most of us become tense when we are under stress, so it is important to learn to release the tension from your body. Practice the muscle relaxation technique below to ease the effects of a tense day. This exercise is beneficial because it is a way to completely relax your body and put your brain at rest.

- Get comfortable in your favorite chair.
- Breathe deeply and concentrate on your body and how it feels as you sit in the chair. Notice any tension in your neck, shoulders or back.
- Continue breathing and concentrating this way for a few minutes.
- Begin to contract your muscles, starting with your toes and feet; keep your muscles contracted for a few seconds and then slowly relax them. Focus on the feeling of contracting and relaxing your muscles.
- Work your way up your body, continuing to contract and relax your muscles as you go from your feet, to your calves, to your thighs, to your stomach, to your buttocks, to your arms and to your neck—ending with your facial muscles.

When you are finished, take a few more deep breaths. You will notice how much tension you have released and how much better you feel.

Exercise 2: Positive Thinking

Many people get into trouble because they end up thinking and worrying about all the negative things that are happening in their lives. The more you focus on the negative, the worse your situation becomes. Here is a short exercise to help pattern your thought processes to a more positive outlook.

- Find a quiet spot.
- Stop what you are doing and identify what is disturbing you.
- Place your hand over your heart to center your emotions.
- Think of a positive, humorous or joyful event, person or place. For the next few minutes, imagine yourself back in that event, or spending time with that person, or being in that place.
- Next, think of something that you absolutely love and cherish, such as a family member or a beloved pet. Focus on that loving feeling for a few minutes.
- Lastly, reflect on something that you are thankful for in your life.

The basic requirements of Step 2 are theoretically one of the easier parts of the SPP program since it only involves sleeping and learning to relax. But don't take it for granted! Sometimes sleep and relaxation are easier said than done. If you are having problems in either area, turn to Chapter 6 for tips.

It is also Step 2 where you are required to work on all your emotional stresses. Seek counseling if needed. You don't have to solve all your issues at once but you must eat well and sleep through the night in order to handle them better.

Notice!

If you are having an unusually difficult time eating and sleeping correctly, or you are eating and sleeping well but are still experiencing problems with mood, energy or chronic symptoms, now is a good time to have your hormone levels checked.

Step 3: Tapering Off Toxic Chemicals or Avoiding Them Completely

Basic Requirement:

- Toxic chemicals should be eliminated in a specific order from worst to best as listed on the following pages. You should be able to get off of these fairly easily but don't try to quit everything at once; switch to a toxic chemical further down the list if it helps you get off a toxic chemical higher on the list. Caffeine is a great substitute for more harmful substances. If you haven't been drinking tea, you may need to start in order to get off of tobacco, alcohol, and refined sugars. Never, under any circumstances, go the other way on this list.
- You should not be on any prescription medication on this plan. An exception is using a drug for "prevention". Discuss with your doctor the best way to stop this type of medication now.

This Step is to be addressed after Steps 1, 2 and 5 as needed. You need to eat well, sleep through the night, have any missing hormones balanced before you work on stopping your toxic chemical intake. You use these chemicals to self-medicate natural chemical imbalances. However, you can work on improving the toxic chemicals you ingest and tapering off of sugar as you work on your daily nutrition habits, but never stop sugar before eating well.

I call a chemical toxic if the body cannot use it to rebuild. This includes refined sugars, alcohol, nicotine, artificial sugars, caffeine and many prescription drugs. These substances accelerate the turnover of chemicals and cells in your body, and therefore; speed up the normal aging process.

Up until now, you've been continuing toxic chemicals in order to self-medicate your way through meal planning and stress manage-

ment. If you have made significant improvements in your nutrition, stress and sleep issues—and hormone issues if needed—it is now time to get off of all those harmful chemicals. The good news is that now that you are eating properly, relaxing and following a good supplement protocol your body doesn't need all these other stimuli.

> *If you have skipped directly to this step, stop now! These toxic chemicals—including the consumption of sugar—are not the underlying cause of your weight problems, and simply stopping them will not cause you to lose weight. However, you may begin to cut way back on all of them at this point as long as you are working to correct your eating, sleeping, stress and hormone problems, too.*

Illicit Drugs

If you are using illicit drugs and can't quit, seek professional help and follow the healing plan.

Tobacco

It is extremely important to get off of tobacco and it should be fairly easy once you are eating well and are managing your stresses better. However, make sure that you are taking N-acetyl cysteine, extra vitamin C and vitamin E while you are still smoking. These supplements will help block some of the damaging effects of tobacco. Nicotine is less harmful than tobacco, so switch to nicotine first. The following suggestions can help you eliminate tobacco.

- Switch to nicotine patches, inhalers, nasal sprays or gum, and then taper off these nicotine products on a predetermined schedule.
- Taper off by decreasing the amount of tobacco products you use on a predetermined schedule.
- Try hypnosis, acupuncture or any other stop-smoking program.

• Use any of the prescription antismoking medications that contain the chemical bupropion hydrochloride.
• Substitute one stimulating lifestyle habit for another that is not as harmful as tobacco, such as drinking caffeinated beverages or overdoing cardiovascular exercises.
• Stop cold turkey.

Alcohol

Once you have worked on your nutrition and stresses, it should be easy for you to stop drinking alcohol. Cut back to the equivalent of three or fewer glasses of wine or three or fewer bottles of beer a week or eliminate alcohol completely. There is no place for hard liquor on this program.

Artificial Sugars

Stop all artificial sugars cold turkey. Use stevia or xylitol if needed, or switch to organic raw honey or blackstrap molasses and taper off them at your own pace. In general, refined sugars are better than artificial sugars. Get off of diet sodas by either drinking caffeinated teas or coffee or by switching to caffeinated waters.

Sugar and Sugary Foods

Your ultimate goal is to cut back as much as you can on your intake of sugary foods. This should be fairly easy for you, as your sweet tooth will improve once you balance out your meals and snacks. Stop all refined sugar products such as candy and sodas now. However, small amounts of real desserts will not break your program. Do not skip eating—*and* do not substitute sugary foods for balanced meals. Instead, use the following suggestions if you have the desire for something sweet.

- If you want to have dessert, eat whole fat real ice cream, organic cheesecake, or any other dessert made with whole ingredients.
- Eat more fruit topped with organic fresh whipping cream or dark unsweetened chocolate.

Additives, Chemicals Preservatives and Other Fake Chemicals

Stop all preservatives, additives, MSG, fake fats, carbohydrate and fat blockers cold turkey.

Caffeine

Caffeine is the least harmful of the toxic chemicals. You may continue a cup or two of coffee or tea indefinitely. Switch from the worst sources (diet sodas) to the best sources (green tea) of caffeine in this order:

Diet sodas

Sodas

Caffeinated waters

Yerba Mate

Coffee

Black tea

Green tea

You should not need to but if you want to wean off of caffeine, try this method:

Start by going to 3/4 caffeine and 1/4 decaffeinated for each caffeinated beverage you normally consume. Do not taper off the number of beverages that you drink in a day. If you do not feel any ill effects after a week, then it is time to cut back to 1/2 caffeine and 1/2 decaffeinated for each beverage. After a week, assuming you feel okay, taper off to 1/4 caffeine and 3/4 decaffeinated for each beverage. You

could be completely off the caffeinated form of this beverage by the fourth week. Do this until you are drinking one to two cups of coffee or tea a day. Then go on to another issue and revisit coming fully off of caffeine another day, month or year.

> *By this time you should be drinking plenty of water to substitute for all the sodas, juices, milk and caffeinated drinks that you have stopped drinking.*

Over-the-Counter Drugs

Stop your OTCs at this point and use the supplements suggested in Chapter 7 instead for whatever ails you.

Prescription Drugs

You should not be taking any prescription drugs for chronic problems. If you are, you should be following the Healing Plan.

Step 4: Smart Exercise

Basic Requirements:

Up to five days a week of strenuous exercise as follows:

- Three times a week on nonconsecutive days: 30 to 60 minutes of adaptive exercise with stretching
- Two times a week on opposite days of adaptive exercises: 30 to 45 of calming exercises and/or stimulating exercises with stretching, your choice.
- You can do calming exercises every day if you so desire

Acceptable Adaptive Exercises:

- Ball and band work
- Core strength exercises/mat classes/calisthenics
- Light weight routine
- Pilates
- Pool exercises
- Yoga (strengthening types of yoga only)

Acceptable Calming Exercises:

- Light stretching
- Restorative yoga (not Bikhram)
- Slow swimming*
- Slow walking*

*Only calming if you keep your heart rate at or below 90 beats a minute the whole time.

Unacceptable Exercises:

- Bikhram yoga
- Running
- Spinning exercise bike classes
- Stair stepper aerobic machines

If you have skipped directly to this step, stop now! Simply starting or changing your exercise routine will not solve your weight issues. You must correct your eating, sleeping, stress and hormone problems first. However, if you are overexercising, you can begin tapering down simultaneously while improving your eating, sleeping and hormone issues.

If you are exercising more than recommended or have not been

exercising at all, don't try to match this workout the first day. Follow the appropriate instructions to help your body adjust to your new routine.

Starting an Exercise Routine

If you are out of shape and over the age of fifty, consult your physician for clearance to exercise. If you have any back, neck or joint problems, always consult your physician before starting any exercise routine.

If you have not been exercising at all, use the adaptive and calming exercises I laid out in Chapter 8. Begin by choosing three exercises from the adaptive program and two from the calming program, doing 12 repetitions of each one. Do this program three times a week, resting one day in between each session. Within two weeks, you should be able to work up to doing 12 repetitions of all 10 exercises three times a week.

As your stamina improves, add slow walking or one of the other acceptable calming exercises for half an hour two times a day on the days that you are not doing your adaptive workout. Don't try to do a lot more than this amount of exercise until you have consistently done this for two to four weeks. Then increase as tolerated to the recommended amount of exercise for this plan.

Never exercise unless you have been eating and sleeping well. You are not going to help your metabolism or lose weight faster if you exercise when you are mentally or physically exhausted. Don't push it. Overexercising will cause you to damage your metabolism.

Do not use this program as an excuse to never exercise. A moderate exercise program is an integral part of the Schwarzbein Principle Program.

Tapering Off of Overexercising

If you are overexercising, you need to taper down the amount of stimulating exercises you are doing as soon as possible. You can do this at your own pace. Switch over as quickly as you can to the prescribed exercise regimen. But remember—you never have to do any stimulating exercises ever again to have a long, healthy and heart-disease free life or your ideal body composition.

If you are in great shape and are eating well and sleeping enough hours at night to handle the extra exercise, it is okay to work out strenuously six days a week. Alternate adaptive and stimulating exercises and never do them on the same day. If you are younger than 35 years old, you can do a 1:1 ratio between these two, i.e., for each hour of adaptive you could do an hour of stimulating but not more! If you are older than 35 but younger than 60, you can do a 1.5:1 ratio, more adaptive than stimulating. If you are older than 60 make sure you are doing a 2:1 adaptive to stimulating program. You can always do more resistance than stimulating but never do it the other way around.

If you are interested in working out with me in the privacy of your own home, I have put together several exercise routines that I offer through my Web site, *www.schwarzbeinprinciple.com.*

Step 5: Hormones

Fixing your hormone issue is the only way to achieve true balance. The only way to know if you have a hormone problem is to have your levels checked. You cannot do this one on your own. Please review Chapter 9 if you know or think you may have a hormone problem. Work with a health professional who understands that all hormone systems are interconnected and that one hormone out of balance means that all your hormones are out of balance.

———————————————————————

Congratulations on making it through the step-by-step program. You have made many life-altering changes to nutrition and lifestyle habits that will keep you healthy, happy and strong. I applaud you.

Conclusion

I hope by now you understand that making the necessary changes to your nutrition and lifestyle habits is a process. Do not get down on yourself. Change takes time. I want you to know that everything you do for yourself that is better than what you did before is contributing to your future health and well-being. Remember that you must be healthy to lose weight, not lose weight to be healthy. You will eventually achieve your ideal body composition if you follow my program, *but your health comes first.* Don't let anyone tell you differently. You now have all the information you need to have a happy, long and disease-free life. I hope you act on it and join the thousands of others who have completed this program before you.

Please visit my Web site, *www.schwarzbeinprinciple.com,* where I have listed the most common questions asked in relation to this program. If you have a straightforward nutrition or lifestyle habit question, please don't hesitate to e-mail my staff at *questions@schwarzbeinprinciple.com*

I wish you all the best today and for always.

Diana Schwarzbein, MD

Appendix A

Protein Requirement Calculations

Follow the instructions provided to come up with a personalized protein range for each day, which will need to be divided between meals and snacks.

Start by finding your ideal weight for your height and gender using the Metropolitan Life Tables for Ideal Body Weight.

If you already fall into the ranges for the ideal body weight for your height and sex, use your current weight rounded off to the nearest five pounds and find your precalculated protein ranges. Divide your total protein intake between your meals and snacks. Most people like to eat larger portions for meal times and less for snacks. However, if you would like, it is perfectly acceptable to eat the same portion sizes at each sitting as long as your total protein requirement is not exceeded.

Protein requirements if you are over or under your ideal weight

If your current weight is not in your ideal body weight range, take your current weight, add it to your ideal body weight (use the weight found in parenthesis) and divide by two. This is your first goal weight and will be your "ideal body weight" for the time being. Round this

number to the nearest five pounds and locate your precalculated protein ranges.

Current weight _____ + ideal body weight (the weight in parenthesis) _____ = _____ ÷ 2 = my first goal weight of _____.

Divide your total protein intake between your meals and snacks. Most people like to eat larger portions of food for meal times and less for snacks. However, if you would like, it is perfectly acceptable to eat the same portion sizes at all sittings as long as your total protein requirement is not exceeded.

When you have reached your first weight goal, repeat these calculations and come up with the next weight goal. Continue this procedure as needed until your current weight falls into the normal ranges for your height. Do not worry if it takes a while to reach your ideal body weight. Healing takes time.

Protein requirements and exercise

You will notice that the amount of protein you require is also dependent on how much exercise you do in the day. See exercise descriptions on the next page to determine which range of protein you will need to follow. Unless you are "addicted" to exercise, everyone who has a damaged metabolism should be in the sedentary to moderately active range category; you can be moderately active if you have a healthy metabolism. If you are exercising at an extremely active level, you need to taper down.

Explanation of Activity Levels

- **Sedentary**—no formal activity to small amounts of calming exercises.
- **Moderately Active**—equivalent to slow daily walking for 30 to 45 minutes and up to 45 minutes of light adaptive exercise three times a week with 30 minutes of calming exercises two times a week.
- **Very Active**—30 to 45 minutes of heavy adaptive exercises three times a week and 20 to 30 minutes of stimulating exercises two times a week. This amount of activity should only be done if you have a healthy metabolism. However, some of you will be doing this amount of activity as self-medication. Until you taper down to a more reasonable amount of exercise, you will need to eat at least 5 to 10 more grams of carbohydrates each time you eat (5 if you have diabetes or the metabolic syndrome and 10 if you don't) and more protein ounces.
- **Extremely Active**—45 to 60 minutes of heavy adaptive exercises three times a week and 45 to 60 minutes of stimulating exercises two times a week. If you have a damaged metabolism you should never be doing this amount of activity. If you are doing this much, you need to taper down to "Very Active" immediately. If you exercise too much, you will never heal.

Metropolitan Life Tables for Ideal Body Weight

WOMEN

Ideal body weight

Height	Small frame	Medium frame	Large frame
4'9"	99-108 (103)	106-118 (112)	115-128 (122)
4'10"	100-110 (105)	108-120 (114)	117-131 (124)
4'11"	101-112 (107)	110-123 (117)	119-134 (127)
5'0"	103-115 (109)	112-126 (119)	122-137 (130)
5'1"	105-118 (111)	116-129 (122)	125-140 (133)
5'2"	108-121 (114)	118-132 (125)	128-144 (136)
5'3"	111-124 (117)	121-135 (128)	131-148 (139)
5'4"	114-127 (120)	124-138 (131)	134-152 (143)
5'5"	117-130 (123)	127-141 (134)	137-156 (146)
5'6"	120-133 (126)	130-144 (137)	140-160 (150)
5'7"	123-136 (129)	133-147 (140)	143-164 (153)
5'8"	126-139 (132)	136-150 (143)	146-167 (156)
5'9"	129-142 (135)	139-153 (146)	149-170 (159)
5'10"	132-145 (138)	142-156 (149)	152-173 (162)
5'11"	135-148 (141)	145-159 (152)	155-176 (165)
6'0"	138-151 (144)	148-162 (155)	158-179 (168)

MEN

Ideal body weight

Height	Small frame	Medium frame	Large frame
5'1"	123-129 (126)	126-136 (131)	133-145 (139)
5'2"	125-131 (128)	128-138 (133)	135-148 (141)
5'3"	127-133 (130)	130-140 (135)	137-151 (144)
5'4"	129-135 (132)	132-143 (137)	139-155 (147)
5'5"	131-137 (134)	134-146 (140)	141-159 (150)
5'6"	133-140 (136)	137-149 (143)	145-163 (154)
5'7"	135-143 (139)	140-152 (146)	147-167 (158)
5'8"	137-145 (142)	143-155 (149)	150-171 (162)
5'9"	139-149 (144)	146-158 (152)	153-175 (166)
5'10"	141-152 (146)	149-161 (155)	156-179 (170)
5'11"	144-155 (148)	152-165 (158)	159-183 (174)
6'0"	147-159 (150)	155-169 (161)	163-187 (178)
6'1"	150-163 (153)	159-173 (165)	167-192 (183)
6'2"	153-167 (156)	162-177 (169)	171-197 (188)
6'3"	157-171 (160)	166-182 (174)	176-202 (193)

Chart of "ideal" weight in pounds and protein range in ounces with different activity levels.

Protein range in ounces (multiply by 7 to get grams)

Weight in Pounds	Sedentary to Moderately Active	Very Active to Extremely Active
100	6.5–8.0	9.75–11.50
105	6.75–8.50	10.0–11.75
110	7.0–9.0	10.5–12.25
115	7.50–9.25	11.25–13.0
120	7.75–9.75	11.75–13.50
125	8.0–10.0	12.0–14.0
130	8.5–10.50	12.75–15.0
135	8.75–11.0	13.0–15.25
140	9.0–11.25	13.50–15.75
145	9.5–11.75	14.25–16.75
150	9.75–12.0	14.75–17.0
155	10.0–12.50	15.0–17.50
160	10.5–13.0	15.75–18.25
165	10.75–13.50	16.25–18.75
170	11.0–13.75	16.50–19.25
175	11.25–14.0	17.0–19.75
180	11.75–14.50	17.75–20.50
185	12.0–15.0	18.0–21.0
190	12.25–15.5	18.5–21.50
195	12.75–15.75	19.25–22.25
200	13.0–16.25	19.5–22.75
205	13.25–16.75	20.0–23.25
210	13.75–17.0	20.75–24.0
215	14.0–17.50	21.0–24.50
220	14.25–17.75	21.50–25.0
225	14.50–18.25	21.75–25.50
230	15.0–18.75	22.50–26.25
235	15.25–19.0	23.0–26.75
240	15.50–19.50	23.25–27.0
245	16.0–20.0	24.0–28.0
250	16.25–20.25	24.50–28.50

Appendix B

Achieving Bowel Health

Some of you have damaged your intestines to the point that you cannot digest your food correctly, you have food allergies, you have damaged the lining of your small intestine so that you don't absorb your food correctly and/or you have an overgrowth of unwanted bacteria or fungus in your large intestine. If you feel you have any of these problems, or if you have an autoimmune disease, chronic constipation, unexplained rashes, irritability, frequent headaches, dark circles under your eyes, excema, irritable bowel syndrome, bloating after you eat, an inability to lose fat weight despite following the Healing Plan correctly or you just don't feel well after three months of your new way of eating, you should try the rotation/elimination meal plans with the phase one supplement recommendations. Remember to chew your food thoroughly and use HCL and/or digestive enzymes as needed.

At this point I recommend that you work with a GI holistic health specialist who believes in and understands food allergies. Please visit my Web site for further recommendations on healing your gastrointestinal tract at *www.schwarzbeinprinciple.com*

25 gram Sample Elimination/Rotation Diet

Basic Guidelines: Eliminate *gluten, soy,* and *cow's milk foods* from your diet for at least 1 month–don't eat eggs more than 2 times a week

(Dairy products from goat, sheep, and buffalo's milk are acceptable)

Rotate all foods as much as possible by eating them once every three days.

Each meal contains approximately 25 grams of carbohydrates

MEALS	MONDAY	TUESDAY	WEDNESDAY	THURSDAY	FRIDAY	SATURDAY	SUNDAY
Breakfast	1 1/2 slices of rice bread w/organic, sugar-free almond butter *carrot sticks	Breakfast Burrito: eggs, avocado slices, chopped tomato wrapped in a large corn tortilla	Nitrate-free turkey sausage 3/4 cup roasted potatoes w/ onions and peppers	Salmon w/ sliced cucumber, dill, and goat cheese on 1 slices rice bread toast	Scrambled eggs Fresh salsa 1/4 cup black beans 1 small corn tortilla	1 cup goat milk yogurt, cinnamon, and chopped walnuts 7 Nut Thin crackers *Celery sticks	Turkey burger patty 2 small baked red potatoes *Sliced tomatoes
Lunch	Grilled salmon spinach salad w/ roasted red peppers, feta crumbles (from goat cheese), 1/2 cup chick peas, and vinaigrette	Buffalo burger topped w/ lettuce, tomato, pickles, and Dijon 2/3 cup lentil soup	Grilled shrimp served on a bed of romaine w/ tomato wedges, green onions, and snap peas served w/ vinaigrette 15 Savory Thins	Chinese Chix Salad: mixed greens, shredded cabbage, grilled chicken, and almond slivers with oil and vinegar 1 small jicama, chopped	Tuna salad made w/ celery and pure pressed oil mayo 13 Edward & Son Brown Rice Snaps *Raw veggies	Fish Tacos: Fish of choice w/ shredded cabbage, tomato, onions, cilantro, sliced avocado, and fresh salsa in 1 medium corn tortilla	Mexican Salad: lettuce, seasoned ground sirloin, 1/2 cup kidney beans, fresh salsa, guacamole
Dinner	Steak smothered w/ sautéed onions, mushrooms, and peppers Small baked potato w/ dab of butter Grilled zucchini Add salad if desired	Grilled chicken 1 large artichoke, steamed dipped in pure pressed oil mayonnaise Mixed green salad w/ Italian dressing	Baked halibut 1 cup butternut squash Green beans and 1/3 cup corn Add salad if desired	Stir-fried pork and vegetables over 1/2 cup buckwheat Mixed green salad w/ vinaigrette	Grilled sea bass Sautéed spinach, garlic, and olive oil 1 small sweet potato w/ dab of butter Chopped cucumber, carrots and tomatoes w/ vinaigrette	Grilled lamb shank 3/4 cup green peas Broccoli and cauliflower mix Add salad as desired	Chicken baked w/ lemon, garlic, olive oil and seasoning served over 1 cup spaghetti squash w/ asparagus spears and sundried tomatoes Add salad as desired

1. When bread is indicated, use: Rice Bread; Crackers: Edward & Son (brown rice snaps), Nut Thins, Black Sesame Seed Rice Crackers (Whole Foods); Tortillas: Corn Dressings: Drew's, Spectrum, Newman's Own Oil & Vinegar and Caesar, Annie's Italian

2. If raw vegetables are indicated, use: carrots, celery, onions, cucumber, broccoli, cauliflower, peppers.

3. Mixed greens could include: variety of lettuce, spinach, tomatoes, grated carrots, cucumber, celery, peppers.

4. When butter is indicated, use organic, raw unsweetened, unsalted butter.

5. If you are a diabetic, raw carrots and tomatoes may cause blood sugar to increase.

30 gram Sample Elimination/Rotation Diet

Basic Guidelines: Eliminate *gluten, soy,* and *cow's milk* foods from your diet for at least 1 month–don't eat eggs more than 2 times a week
(Dairy products from goat, sheep, and buffalo's milk are acceptable)
Rotate all foods as much as possible by eating them once every three days.

Each meal contains approximately 30 grams of carbohydrates

MEALS	MONDAY	TUESDAY	WEDNESDAY	THURSDAY	FRIDAY	SATURDAY	SUNDAY
Breakfast	2 slices of rice bread w/organic, sugar-free almond butter *carrot sticks	Breakfast Burrito: eggs, avocado slices, chopped tomato wrapped in a large corn tortilla	Nitrate-free turkey sausage 1 cup roasted potatoes w/ onions and peppers	Salmon w/ sliced cucumber, dill, and goat cheese on 2 slices rice bread toast	Scrambled eggs Fresh salsa 1/3 cup black beans 1 small corn tortilla	1 cup goat milk yogurt, cinnamon, and chopped walnuts 10 Nut Thins *Celery sticks	Turkey burger patty 2 small baked red potatoes *Sliced tomatoes
Lunch	Grilled salmon spinach salad w/ roasted red peppers, feta crumbles (from goat cheese), 1/3 cup chick peas, 1/3 cup navy beans, and vinaigrette	Buffalo burger topped w/lettuce, tomato, pickles, and Dijon 3/4 cup lentil soup	Grilled shrimp served on a bed of romaine w/ tomato wedges, green onions, and snap peas served w/ vinaigrette 18 Savory Thins	Chinese Chix Salad: mixed greens, shredded cabbage, grilled chicken, and almond slivers with oil and vinegar 1 medium jicama, chopped	Tuna salad made w/ celery and pure pressed oil mayo 16 Edward & Son Brown Rice Snaps *Raw veggies	Fish Tacos: Fish of choice w/ shredded cabbage, tomato, onions, cilantro, sliced avocado, and fresh salsa in 2 small corn tortillas	Mexican Salad: lettuce, seasoned ground sirloin, 1/2 cup kidney beans, fresh salsa, guacamole
Dinner	Steak smothered w/ sautéed onions, mushrooms, and peppers Medium baked potato w/ dab butter Grilled zucchini Add salad if desired	Grilled chicken 1 large artichoke, steamed dipped in pure pressed oil mayonnaise 1/3 cup quinoa Mixed green salad w/ Italian dressing	Baked halibut 1 cup butternut squash Green beans and 1/3 cup corn Add salad if desired	Stir-fried pork and vegetables over 2/3 cup buckwheat Mixed green salad w/ vinaigrette	Grilled sea bass Sautéed spinach, garlic, and olive oil 1 medium sweet potato w/ dab butter Chopped cucumber, carrots and tomatoes w/vinaigrette	Grilled lamb shank 1 cup lima beans Broccoli and cauliflower mix Add salad as desired	Chicken baked w/lemon, garlic, olive oil and seasoning served over 1 cup spaghetti squash w/asparagus spears, 1/3 cup peas, and sundried tomatoes Add salad as desired

1. When bread is indicated, use: Rice Bread; Crackers: Edward & Son (brown rice snaps), Nut Thins, Black Sesame Seed Rice Crackers (Whole Foods); Tortillas: Corn Dressings: Drew's, Spectrum, Newman's Own Oil & Vinegar and Caesar, Annie's Italian

2. If raw vegetables are indicated, use: carrots, celery, onions, cucumber, broccoli, cauliflower, peppers.

3. Mixed greens could include: variety of lettuce, spinach, onions, tomatoes, grated carrots, cucumber, celery, peppers.

4. When butter is indicated, use organic, raw unsweetened, unsalted butter.

Gluten-Free Diet

You will be following a gluten free diet if you are on the first few months of the Healing Plan, have a known gluten intolerance, are following one of the rotation/elimination plans or have not improved after three months of the Maintenance nutrition plan. Do not despair, you still have plenty of foods to eat!

Foods To Avoid That Contain Gluten

The following grains, including their flours all contain gluten. You must avoid them while following a gluten free diet.

Wheat	Couscous	Spelt
Barley	Durum flour	Semolina
Bran	Kamut	Triticale
Bulgar	Rye	

Hidden Sources Of Gluten

Please read food labels of all processed foods for the following ingredients that contain gluten.

Modified food starch (if contains wheat)

Dextrin (unless noted as corn or tapioca dextrin)

Flavorings and extracts (often made from a gluten-containing grain alcohol)

Hydrolyzed vegetable protein (some are made using wheat)

Imitation seafood (may include wheat as a binding agent)

Creamed or thickened products such as soups, stews and sauces, unless homemade

Exceptions

- Oats—Avoid if you have full-blown celiac disease, but try eating oats if you only have gluten intolerance. Make sure to eat

packaged oats, not those found in bins as they can be cross cont-
aminated with wheat products.

- You may be able to tolerate sourdough bread, but you are not
  allowed to try this until you have been gluten free for at least three
  months on the Healing Plan and after six months if you know you
  have a gluten intolerance.

Foods Allowed

Amaranth	Corn	Potato
Arrowroot	Jicama	Rice
Artichoke	Lentils	Squash
Beans	Lima beans	Sweet potato
Buckwheat	Millet	Yams
Chick peas	Peas	
Cooked carrots/tomatoes	All other starchy vegetables, too	

Where To Shop For Gluten-Free Foods

Your local health food store
Trader Joe's
Whole foods

Web Sites:

Note: Many food products sold on these web sites may not be suit-
able for you due to high sugar content; pick and choose carefully.

glutensolutions.com for food products
glutenfreepantry.com for food products, mixes, and recipes
livingwithout.com for gluten free info., recipes, and tips. Their
   magazine is called *Living Without*.
gfcdiet.com for useful information on the gluten free, casein free diet

Dairy-Restricted Diet

If you are allergic to dairy, you are allergic to casein, the protein found in cow's milk. You will need to read labels (ingredient lists) carefully because casein may be hidden in many foods. If you have a gluten intolerance, you may also have a casein intolerance. If you don't feel well on a gluten free plan, follow the gluten and dairy free guidelines together. Being allergic to casein is not the same thing as being lactose intolerant. If you are lactose intolerant, you are unable to digest milk sugar causing bloating, cramping and loose bowel movements. However, you can have both a casein allergy and be lactose intolerant.

Foods to Avoid

- Cow's milk
- Cheese—Avoid all cheeses made from cow's milk
- Yogurt—Avoid all yogurt made from cow's milk
- Sour cream (cow's milk)
- Cream cheese (cow's milk)
- Ice cream (cow's milk)

Dairy Foods Allowed

- Organic, whole-fat whipping cream*
- Organic, unsalted butter*
- Goat's milk products**—goat cheese, goat's milk yogurt
- Sheep's milk products**—Feta cheese, Roquefort cheese (monitor saturated fat), any sheep milk cheeses
- Buffalo mozzarella**

———————————

*Use cream and butter moderately because they both contain small amounts of casein. Avoid completely if you are very allergic to casein.

**In general goat, sheep and buffalo dairy does not contain casein. Unfortunately, manufacturers of these products may add casein to their products. Read labels very carefully.

Snack Ideas
Without Gluten, Cow's Dairy & Soy
25 grams Carbohydrates

- 1½ cup whole strawberries and goat cheese
- 2 slices of gluten free bread (25g) and organic sugar-free peanut butter
- 5 Corn Thins with egg salad, tuna salad, or chicken salad
- 1 small baked potato with buffalo mozzarella cheese and fresh salsa
- 4 cups air popped popcorn and mixed nuts
- 1½ cup raspberries and sunflower seeds
- 1 slice rice, buckwheat, or millet bread (25g) with ¼ avocado, and chicken salad
- 1 cup organic, plain, goat milk yogurt, ½ cup blueberries, and crushed walnuts
- 2 slices gluten free bread (25g), tomatoes, feta cheese, and carrot sticks
- 18 Nut Thin crackers with almond butter
- 1 slice rice bread (25g), nitrate free turkey, lettuce, tomato, and mayonnaise (canola base)
- 1 small sweet potato and nitrate free chicken sausage
- 13 Edward & Son brown rice snaps, cucumber, and goat cheese
- 2 small corn tortillas (25g), melted buffalo mozzarella cheese, avocado, and fresh salsa
- 1 small grapefruit and hard boiled egg(s)
- ½ cup hummus, 5 Nut Thin crackers, raw vegetables, and cashews
- 16 Nut Thin crackers, buffalo mozzarella cheese, and spicy mustard

To round out your snacks, add some non-starchy vegetables such as celery, carrots, tomatoes, cucumbers, peppers, broccoli, snap peas, and cauliflower.

Snack Ideas
Without Gluten, Cow's Dairy & Soy
30 grams Carbohydrates

- 2 cups whole strawberries and goat cheese
- 1 to 2 slices of gluten free bread or crackers (30g) and organic sugar-free peanut butter
- 6 Corn Thins with egg salad, tuna salad, or chicken salad
- 1 medium baked potato with buffalo mozzarella cheese and fresh salsa
- 4½ cups air popped popcorn and mixed nuts
- 1½ cup blackberries and sunflower seeds
- 1 slice rice, buckwheat, or millet bread (30g) with ¼ avocado, and chicken salad
- 1 cup organic, plain, goat milk yogurt, ½ cup blueberries, and crushed walnuts
- 1 slice gluten free bread (30g), tomatoes, feta cheese, and carrot sticks
- 23 Nut Thin crackers with almond butter
- 1 slice rice bread (30g), nitrate free turkey, lettuce, tomato, and mayonnaise (pure pressed oils)
- 1 medium sweet potato and nitrate free chicken sausage
- 23 Nut Thin crackers, buffalo mozzarella cheese, and spicy mustard
- 16 Edward & Son brown rice snaps, cucumber, and goat cheese
- 2 small corn tortillas (30g), melted buffalo mozzarella cheese, avocado, and fresh salsa
- 1 medium grapefruit and hard boiled egg(s)
- ½ cup hummus, 10 Nut Thin crackers, raw vegetables, and cashews

To round out your snacks, add some non-starchy vegetables such as celery, carrots, tomatoes, cucumbers, peppers, broccoli, snap peas, and cauliflower.

Supplements for Digestive Health

If you have food allergies, you probably also have some inflamma-tion in your GI tract due to the allergic reaction. The way to get rid of this inflammation is to avoid all the foods that you are allergic to and take these supplements that are designed to decrease the inflamma-tion and help heal the lining of your intestines that may have been damaged from your allergic reaction.

Anti-inflammatory Supplements

Please read the ingredients of these supplements and stop any of your usual supplements that overlap with this regimen, Start these supplements first to help calm your intestines by decreasing inflammation.

- Bio-Inflammatory Plus Shake   2 scoops/shake
                                     2 shakes/day in place of
                                     meals or snacks

Mix into shake:
- Intestinal Repair Complex   1 rounded teaspoon x 2 shakes
- MSM powder (1t=5000 mg MSM) 1rounded teaspoon x 2 shakes
- Omega Marine Liquid   1 teaspoon x 2 shakes
  (1t=1500 mg EPA/DHA)
- OptiFiber   1/2 scoop x 2 shakes

  Or

- Bio-Inflammatory Plus Shake   same as above

Mix into shake to make a "Gut Goo":
- Organic applesauce   1/2 cup
- Freshly ground Flax Meal   1 to 2 teaspoons
- Glutamine Powder   1 tablespoon
- Plain MSM powder   1 teaspoon

Take separately:
- Betaine HCl   See below for instructions
- Three a day Antioxidant   1 pill with all meals

In one month, add these supplements:
- Digestive Enzymes   1-2 before meals and snacks
- Probiotics (healthy bacteria to   Take as directed
  re-colonize your colon)

Betaine Hydrochloride Instructions

Note: If you have heartburn or acid reflux, do NOT take Betaine HCl. If you do not display any symptoms of heartburn, follow the directions listed below to optimize therapy for digestive health.

Instructions:

Start by taking Week 1 dose. Increase supplementation every week, as instructed below, until you start to display heartburn symptoms. Once you experience acid reflux or heartburn, follow the protocol from the previous week when you did not have any symptoms.

Week 1:
1 pill with meals
1 pill with snacks

Week 3:
2 pills with meals
2 pills with snacks

Week 2:
2 pill with meals
1 pill with snacks

Week 4:
3 pills with meals
2 pills with snacks

Taking Betaine HCl with digestive enzymes will further enhance digestion. Once instructed to start digestive enzymes, take 2 pills with meals and 1-2 with snacks.

About the Author

Diana Schwarzbein, MD, is a leading authority on metabolic healing. She graduated from the University of Southern California (USC) Medical School and completed her residency in internal medicine and a fellowship in endocrinology at the Los Angeles County USC Medical Center.

Dr. Schwarzbein's first book, *The Schwarzbein Principle* (with Nancy Deville) laid out the ideas behind her revolutionary approach to health. It became a publishing phenomenon, selling more than 250,000 copies and changing countless lives for the better. Her other books include *The Schwarzbein Principle II: The Transition* (with Marilyn Brown), *The Schwarzbein Principle Cookbook,* and *The Schwarzbein Principle Vegetarian Cookbook.*

In addition to her private practice, Dr. Schwarzbein lectures frequently on diabetes, weight loss, metabolism, menopause, and related subjects. She lives with her husband in Santa Barbara, California.

www.schwarzbeinprinciple.com.